NUR

FOR PATIENT-CENTERED CARE

Authenticity Presence Intuition Expertise

Senada,
I have heard this text is imperative to any new nursing leader. Congratulations on a successfully managed very first survey. I hope it gives you the motivation and drive to push through the challenges in your role.
Until we get to collaborate again!
  —Derek M.

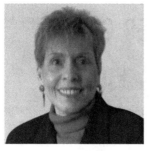

Harriet Forman, EdD, RN, is a well-known nurse leader, educator, published author, and editor of the Cherry Ames series of books. She is a specialist in communication, management and leadership development, redesign, and patient-centered care and team building as critical components of patient and staff satisfaction and retention. She has been a chief nurse executive of both acute and long-term care facilities and worked with *Nursing Spectrum* in various executive and editorial positions, including launching the New York/New Jersey division, serving as executive director for the Florida division, and fulfilling corporate executive and editorial responsibilities. She also participated in launching what is now *Healthcare Traveler* magazine. Dr. Forman coauthored a labor relations column published over a 2.5-year time period in *Journal of Nursing Administration,* as well as many professional articles and a chapter on collective bargaining in *Leadership and Nursing Care Management* edited by Dr. Diane Huber.

Her previous experience comprises both clinical and administration. Dr. Forman's teaching practice includes adjunct graduate faculty lecturing at several universities and continuing education instruction to groups as large as 1,200 participants. She is widely published and is a member of nursing and health care leadership-related organizations including Sigma Theta Tau. Dr. Forman has been accepted as a National Labor Relations Board expert witness in labor relations and managerial communications and as a Florida federal court expert witness in nursing administration. She worked internationally with health care, nursing, and medical personnel in Russia and addressed the first Congress of the All Russian Nurses Association in Saint Petersburg. She is a board member and senior consultant for The Center To Promote Health Care Studies, a Distinguished Alumnus of The Mount Sinai Hospital School of Nursing Alumni Association, and has her professional collection archived at the Center for Nursing History, Guilderland, NY, on invitation from the Foundation of the New York State Nurses Association. Her education ranges from a diploma in nursing from The Mount Sinai Hospital School of Nursing to a Doctorate in Education with a focus on the Nurse Executive Role from Columbia University Teachers College.

Foreword by Deborah M. Tascone
Deborah M. Tascone, RN, MS, is regional executive director of the North Shore-Long Island Jewish Health System located in the New York City metropolitan area.

She is responsible for multiple acute care hospitals within the system. Ms. Tascone joined the health system as a nurse director in 1995 and was the first registered nurse and first woman to be appointed as a hospital executive director. Prior to that, she was employed in various health-related positions, applying her clinical background to the development of new programs and services throughout the hospitals for which she is responsible.

Ms. Tascone is a member of the American College of Healthcare Executives and is the president of the board of directors of Project REAL (Residential Experience in Adult Living). She has been a guest speaker for Healthcare America's conference: Customer Service for the Healthcare Industry, where she presented on the topic "Healthcare Reform: Leadership from the Front Lines." She has also guest lectured at Sweden's Helsingborg Hospital and Uppsala University on the role of the CEO in the integrated health care system. In 2007, she attended the World Health Executive Forum in Montreal, Canada, where international health care leaders and government officials discussed "Strategic Health Issues—Global Vision."

Ms. Tascone epitomizes a patient-centered health care professional who is well-known for her intuitive, empathetic staff and patient relationships.

Prologue by Patricia Munhall

Patricia Munhall, EdD, ARNP, PsyA, FAAN, is a Fellow of the American Academy of Nursing and a former professor of nursing and nurse administrator in several universities from New York to Miami, Florida, has concurrently been in practice as a psychoanalyst. She received her doctorate in nursing from Columbia University and graduated from the Academy of Clinical and Applied Psychoanalysis. She is an international speaker on phenomenology as a research method, psychoanalysis, and human understanding. Dr. Munhall is also an author or editor of 11 books and over 70 manuscripts and chapters focusing on qualitative research, unknowing, phenomenology, and philosophical analysis. The latest is the fifth edition of *Nursing Research: A Qualitative Perspective.*

Dr. Munhall is founder and President of the International Institute for Human Understanding, headquartered in Miami, Florida. The Institute, a not-for-profit organization, exists to foster compassion, tolerance, and justice (www.iihu.org). In addition to her other works, Dr. Munhall consults for qualitative research and speaks on phenomenology at workshops and conferences, and she engages in continuous active publishing on qualitative research methods. She currently resides in Miami where she has a full-time practice as a nurse practitioner and psychoanalyst.

Chapter 7 by Barbara Stevens Barnum

Barbara Stevens Barnum, PhD, RN, FAAN, is a noted presence in nursing education. She is the author of 11 books—many with numerous editions—with chapters in many other titles (five published by Springer), and of countless peer-reviewed articles. She has served as editor, *Nursing Leadership Forum* (Springer) and editor, *Nursing & Health Care*, NLN (the previous incarnation of NLN's *Nursing Education Perspectives*). She is currently a consultant, psychotherapist, and part-time faculty and periodic lecturer at NYU College of Nursing. Previous positions include director, Division of Health Services, Sciences and Education, Teachers College, Columbia University, New York, where she also held the Stewart Chair and chair in the Department of Nursing Education. She was a consultant at Columbia-Presbyterian Medical Center, New York, and her first academic position was as professor, Nursing Administration, College of Nursing, University of Illinois, Chicago.

A Fellow of the American Academy of Nursing, Dr. Barnum has worked extensively, both nationally and internationally, as a continuing education instructor and consultant, including an 8-year term as consultant to the U. S. Air Force Surgeon General. Dr. Barnum presents workshops in areas of complementary medicine and spirituality nationwide.

NURSING LEADERSHIP FOR PATIENT-CENTERED CARE

Authenticity Presence Intuition Expertise

Harriet Forman, EdD, RN

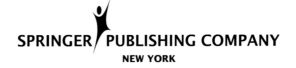

SPRINGER PUBLISHING COMPANY
NEW YORK

Springer Publishing Company, LLC
11 West 42nd Street
New York, NY 10036
www.springerpub.com

Acquisitions Editor: Allan Graubard
Production Editor: Gayle Lee
Cover Design: Steven Pisano
Composition: The Manila Typesetting Company

ISBN: 978-0-8261-0558-5
E-book ISBN: 978-0-8261-0559-2

12 13/ 5 4 3 2

The author and the publisher of this Work have made every effort to use sources believed to be reliable to provide information that is accurate and compatible with the standards generally accepted at the time of publication. Because medical science is continually advancing, our knowledge base continues to expand. Therefore, as new information becomes available, changes in procedures become necessary. We recommend that the reader always consult current research and specific institutional policies before performing any clinical procedure. The author and publisher shall not be liable for any special, consequential, or exemplary damages resulting, in whole or in part, from the readers' use of, or reliance on, the information contained in this book. The publisher has no responsibility for the persistence or accuracy of URLs for external or third-party Internet Web sites referred to in this publication and does not guarantee that any content on such Web sites is, or will remain, accurate or appropriate.

Library of Congress Cataloging-in-Publication Data
Forman, Harriet.
  Nursing leadership for patient-centered care : authenticity, presence, intuition, expertise / Harriet Forman.
    p. ; cm.
  Includes bibliographical references and index.
  ISBN 978-0-8261-0558-5 (alk. paper)—ISBN 978-0-8261-0559-2 (e-book)
  1. Nursing services—Administration. 2. Leadership. 3. Nurse and patient. I. Title.
    [DNLM: 1. Leadership. 2. Nursing. 3. Nurse Administrators. 4. Patient-Centered Care—organization & administration. WY 105]
  RT89.F59 2010
  362.17'3068—dc22

                                                                              2010026538

Special discounts on bulk quantities of our books are available to corporations, professional associations, pharmaceutical companies, health care organizations, and other qualifying groups.

If you are interested in a custom book, including chapters from more than one of our titles, we can provide that service as well.

For details, please contact:
Special Sales Department
Springer Publishing Company, LLC
11 West 42nd Street, 15th Floor
New York, NY 10036-8002
Phone: 877–687–7476 or 212–431–4370
Fax: 212–941–7842
E-mail: sales@springerpub.com

Printed in the United States of America by Gasch Printing.

Contents

NOTE: CNE—Chief Nurse Executive: The author recognizes that it is unlikely that the chief nurse executive will be the individual to lead the many activities this position is depicted as personally directing and controlling. The reader is invited to substitute any management team member for CNE as appropriate to the individual organization.

Vignettes

Foreword

REFORMING PATIENT CARE FROM THE BEDSIDE

I have been blessed to practice nursing for over 30 years. The profession has been a gift that I have embraced with open arms. It has afforded me the ability and opportunity to ease the suffering of others, nurture wonderful friendships, and experience the stability and spirituality of who I am. This devotion also brings with it commitment and responsibility as a patient advocate—never turning away from what we nurses believe is right and never compromising patient care for politics or self interest. I have often said that the day I fail to hear a patient's call bell or request for assistance will be the day that I can no longer call myself a nurse.

First as a staff nurse and then as a nurse leader at various management and administration levels, I have seen nurses become better educated and better paid than ever before. But often drugs and supplies are not available to them when and where they need them. They spend precious time and energy running to pharmacy and to central supply. Often they also have to transport patients instead of providing and directing patient-centered care. Nurses also face the challenge of duplicative paperwork, excessive mandatory meetings, and burgeoning regulations and responsibilities.

At the same time, all too many patients and potential patients speak of hospital experiences with apprehension. Hospital-acquired infections and other iatrogenic conditions are of concern, nursing shortages and the uninsured make headlines, emergency centers overflow, and disgruntled staff members cause labor/management unrest.

Health care reform has occupied the hearts, minds, and halls of congress—seemingly forever. But another kind of health care reform is also needed—in how care is delivered at the bedside.

Among the problems to be solved are impractical nurse/patient ratios; unanswered call bells, especially on nights and weekends; redundant efforts; task orientation; ineffective communication; shifting priorities; managers drawn away from patient-centered care by administrative duties; and tension between and among staff from different cultures. These and other issues impact negatively on both the staff and patient experience, as well as on outcomes.

In her book, *Nursing Leadership for Patient-Centered Care*, Dr. Forman approaches these issues not as an outsider looking to place blame, but as a nurse executive who appreciates nursing and its practitioners—as a nurse-oriented consultant and a nurse leader who has applied practical approaches to improve situations inimical to both patients and staff alike. She leads from within—from a patient-centered, empathetic perspective that allows the manager to *feel* what it is like to live the experience of staff and patient. I know this to be true of her from personal experience—from having worked with and been mentored by her.

Dr. Forman's book is revolutionary and courageous in that it brings to light negative issues that exist in nursing management and patient care. Without change, these will only worsen.

From the first chapter to the last, Dr. Forman cites actual examples that demonstrate such things as a nurse turning her back on a patient with a bleeding wound saying, "I can't intervene without MD's orders." Or of nurses concerning themselves with pedantic rules rather than patients' comfort, racial and religious prejudice causing fulminating hatred that spills out into the patient care arena, favoritism influencing promotions and discipline, and power and authority being abused and misused.

Dr. Forman's work is steeped in theory. She steps outside traditional avenues of study and delves into ancient philosophy, existential psychology, and other intellectual learning realms. She captures readers' imagination and expands their horizons to help them understand their staff members' and patients' life experiences.

The born leader theory takes a prominent position, along with a focus on the magnetism of charisma as a driving force of leadership. She shows us how we can learn from such notable figures as Christ and Gandhi. Among the other theories she draws from are communication theory, leader be-havior style, motivational theory, critical thinking, personality theory, philosophy, ethical decision making, collective bargaining, power and authority, management, leadership, and the organization. Importantly, Dr. Forman's approach is effective application of theory to practice.

Dr. Forman has captured the very essence of the problems that are holding back the patient-centered relationships of nurses, nurse managers, and the interdisciplinary team. Her use of plain day-to-day language and methods will ultimately bring reform to health care at the bedside—where it is essential to the lives of those we serve. This book has the potential to revolutionize nursing management and patient-centered nursing care with the most honest appraisal of what is actually transpiring in many of our centers of care.

Through the examples of breakdowns in care and frank discussion, Dr. Forman describes and dissects common problems. She then reconstructs a stronger, sturdier patient-centered model—one that will withstand scrutiny and the sands of time.

Why this book is essential for every nurse manager and aspiring nurse manager to read: Nursing Leadership for Patient-Centered Care is a page turner. Reading this book, nurses may have *Aha!* moments. It should be thoughtfully read and carefully considered. The ideas put forth need to be discussed: staff and management should be mentored and given time and opportunity to grow, develop, and give personal tension and prejudice the light of day without fear of criticism.

None of this can be done overnight. As we know from trying to reform the greater health care program in the country—true reform takes time, effort, support, consensus, and commitment. Dr. Forman has drawn the new paradigm. Her organizational chart is concentric—the patient is at the center. Now it is up to dedicated nurse managers, leaders, and academics to make it a reality.

Deborah M. Tascone, MS, RN

Acknowledgments

With gratitude, I acknowledge the individuals listed below. Without their influence, I probably would not have been able to write this book. I apologize to those I may have inadvertently omitted.

Allan Graubard—executive editor, Springer Publishing Company. When I brought my idea for this book to Allan, he had the vision and the courage to see merit in a new way to tell an old story. I owe to Allan a world of thanks for advancing my proposal to the publisher.

Florence VanKeuren, MS, RN—former executive director, Visiting Nurse Association of Long Island. I came to her with no applicable clinical experience. Nevertheless, she recognized my potential and employed me; she identified my propensity to function independently; she assigned me accordingly and set me on my life's path.

Sonya Hirschberg, MS, RN—former director of nursing who took a leap of faith and placed me in an administrative position, then mentored me in labor relations and management. She taught me that it was okay to sidestep regulations to serve the greater good.

Rachel Rotkovitch, MS, RN, FAAN—former CNE who understood and used power in creative ways. Although I never worked *for* her, I learned an enormous amount *from* her. Without her personal reference, I would not have landed my next job—as director of nursing at a large, complex medical center in Brooklyn.

Margaret McClure, EdD, RN, FAAN—professor, former CNE, and author of *Magnet Hospitals: Attraction and Retention of Professional Nurses*. Maggie, as she is fondly known, mentored me in several important labor relations areas that I had not yet encountered. She also helped me appreciate the inherent power of time and the fine art of persuasion.

Suzanne Smith, EdD, RN, FAAN—editor-in-chief, *Journal of Nursing Administration (JONA)* and **Leah Curtin, ScD(h), RN, FAAN**—former editor *Nursing Management*; founder *CurtinCalls*; editor emeritus *American Nurse*. Truth be told, I dreaded what they did but appreciated the effect it had upon me. Both of these professional writers/editors took pen in hand and scrupulously edited my early works.

Kevin W. Smyth—founding publisher, *Nursing Spectrum*, who employed me to start the New York/New Jersey division of *Nursing Spectrum*.

Within a few weeks, he taught me what I needed to know about bulk mailing, type setting, printing, and all the myriad details of magazine production and sales to produce a nursing publication. I stayed with the company for 12 years, during which time I met the next person to whom I give thanks.

Robert Wells—who entrusted me with the copyright to the Cherry Ames series of nurse books written by his sister Helen Wells. My mission was to return these books to the marketplace to make them available to nostalgic past readers and, importantly, to today's young readers. Thanks to Springer Publishing, these books are "for sale."

My parents **Frances and Herman Schulman**—who taught me fairness and love of humankind. They raised me in an environment rich with music, poetry, literature, and charitable giving. This established a basis for my pursuing a career in the healing art of nursing—and in writing and publishing.

Joseph (Rsh) Rosenman and Meryl Tihanyi—my son and daughter, who both still try to teach me patience. Funny how as the years go by, roles reverse, and the teacher becomes the student and the student the teacher. Empathy runs deep in them both. I like to think they got that from me.

Sol Forman—listed last but certainly not least—my dear husband: always encouraging, never unwilling to toss around ideas with me, my first and last reader, and the person I count upon to edit out my vestigial purple prose.

Introduction

As you prepare to commit some of your precious time to reading *Nursing Leadership for Patient-Centered Care*, you might want to know something about me—its author. So allow me to introduce myself.

First and foremost, I am a nurse who loves my profession. I have cared for and advocated for patients and for nurses and our line of work throughout a long and fruitful career. During this time, I launched the New York/New Jersey division of *Nursing Spectrum* and served in several corporate editorial and administrative leadership positions. I also helped start *Healthcare Traveler*—a publication for traveling health care professionals.

Before that, I was a chief nurse executive of acute and long-term care facilities, adjunct professor and continuing education instructor, author, and consultant in the United States and in Russia. During these years I conducted innumerable conferences and have spoken with professional nurses in many specialties and at all levels of education and experience. Patients, members of the nursing and the interdisciplinary team, and others in hospitals and long-term care facilities shared their knowledge, opinions, outlook, and recommendations with me.

They have told me many stories. Some have been about wonderful care—about nursing interventions that have saved lives, brought comfort to the dying, and joy to the living. But there are dismaying stories, too, of unnecessary deaths due to inadequate follow-up by nursing supervisors, physicians who did not believe nurses reporting patients in danger, and nurses who did not believe support staff telling of similar events. I have heard of comatose patients aspirating because of poor positioning, and pressure injuries eroding flesh and bone of patients on one-on-one care in ICUs. I have listened to narratives from patients awaiting drugs to ameliorate excruciating pain while nursing staff and pharmacists debated drug delivery responsibility.

During my adjunct faculty experience, I interacted with nurses in the relative quiet of the classroom where ideas could take wing and develop. But students in a classroom—and many of their professors—cannot relate to what it is like to practice in the often hectic environment of the health care delivery setting, where hundreds of patients require care during a hurricane, blizzard, strike, or some other unexpected event that tests the planning, implementation abilities, and mettle of leadership, management, and staff.

Throughout my peripatetic experiences, I observed many things and listened carefully to both people who received care and provided care. As an administrator, or a consultant applying research to practice, I led change from more traditional, ubiquitous hierarchical or matrix models of care to patient-centered versions. There, iatrogenic patient breakdowns such as contractures, shearing and pressure injuries, and hospital-acquired infections were cause for concern long before Medicare imposed reimbursement penalties for such conditions. Our motto was "if we can cure them, we could have prevented them in the first place."

As I spoke to literally thousands of health care professionals and visited health care organizations—acute, long-term, voluntary, proprietary, university-based, and community-based—the same essential factors began to stand out. These are described below, and they are the factors upon which I have based this book.

Essential Factors

1. Empathy—the ability to walk a mile in the shoes of another—be it subordinate staff, peers, and especially patients, was glaringly deficient, especially where hierarchies and intercultural prejudice prevailed. Philosophically, and in practice, there was an absence of sensitivity to others' hurt feelings because of pecking orders, which resulted in the will to "get back." This resulted in labor unrest, collective or insidious reactiveness, and other negative types of lateral or downward violence.

2. The three Cs—collaboration, cooperation, and communication—were not regularly practiced between and among nurses and other entities within the health care setting. Patient-centered care was consequentially fleeting. As an example, nurses and nursing personnel were often out of synch with each other. Instead, there was rivalry and lack of mutual respect among nursing team members as well as between nurses and physicians. A philosophy known as phenomenology—whereby an individual places oneself in another's position and asks how it *feels* to be that person (e.g., patient or a subordinate staff member)—was often absent from the patient-care setting, where egocentricity seemed to be the norm.

3. Patients and patient care were not the center of attention, despite mission and goal statements that identified them as such. Job descriptions were road maps to form and function that sometimes circumscribed and limited action. This often resulted in "It's not my job syndrome." Organizational charts were hierarchical with power and communication flowing from the top down. This led to breakdowns in communication and cooperation. Importantly, nurse managers—middle and upper— were "visibly absent" from patient care areas—some were completely unknown to staff. Few practiced dynamic *management by wandering around* (MBWA). Much time was wasted at meetings and on office work. In many cases, punitive management methods prevailed. There were hierarchies in which relationships between entry-level staff and RNs were damaging to lower-level employees' egos and therefore to patient-centered care.

4. Effective labor relations. *Adversarial relationships are detrimental to patient-centered care.* Management should fully understand their labor agreements and not breach its tenets. In many cases, management personnel had not even seen a labor agreement. They were often intimidated and browbeaten by aggressive union delegates. Sometimes they developed and held grudges against their own staff members long after they had participated in a labor action against their organization. Proper handling of grievances and discipline, performance appraisals, anecdotal records, and other concerns that impacted personnel issues was sorely lacking. Sometimes the notion of making the union a partner in patient-centered care was thought of as a novel idea rather than a goal.

5. Cultural and religious differences needed to be bridged. Favoritism based on race, creed, and national origin was evidenced by supervisory personnel. This often resulted in unfair scheduling and promotion practices. Also, there was intolerance and sometimes palpable hatred among staff members and toward patients. To complicate matters, patients and visitors sometimes demonstrated bigotry toward staff members who were not counseled in handling this appropriately. The need for education and mentoring in dealing with this complex issue from all aspects was compellingly clear.

6. Individuals were being assigned to responsibilities, tasks, and positions with little or no thought to personality traits. For example, "adventurers"

were skipped over for exciting new challenges and "homebodies" were selected to float. This frequently led to negative satisfaction levels, belligerent behavior, poor team building, and unsuccessful outcomes. Patient-centered care and individual staff members suffered and reacted negatively as a result. Management staff failed to understand the reason for unrest and lack of success.

7. Critical thinking, ethical decision making, morality, and power and authority all required further attention. When confronted with complex problems, many individuals seemed ill equipped to take the intellectual steps necessary to reach long-lasting solutions. Ethical decision making appeared to be linked to an individual's personality rather than to ethics as a scholarly matter. People had difficulty separating morality from legality. There was little time to spend on formal education regarding these important issues, and mentoring opportunities were unrecognized. Power and authority were too often misused and abused, thus making full circle back to issues of ethics, morality, and critical thinking.

8. Spirituality—handled therapeutically in that nurse, patient, and manager were at same levels of spiritual development—was rare. Chapter 7, "Spirituality and Nursing: Challenges, Dilemmas, and Occasional Successes," is contributed by a noted researcher in the field: Barbara Stevens Barnum, PhD, RN, FAAN.

9. Grief—the deeply human response to suffering and loss—could have been better handled, whether it was exhibited by a patient or a staff member. Sometimes it was ignored; sometimes it was intellectualized; sometimes personal belief systems were imposed upon others despite resistance. Sometimes it was assuaged with grace and comfort. The bottom line is, I saw it often enough to include it in this book as part of a trilogy: cultural issues, spirituality, and grief. Because in the world of illness and health I have traversed, grief has gone hand-in-hand with life in all its permutations.

10. The term nursing itself needed to be more clearly defined. If you ask nurses what they do, rarely will they say, "I save lives" or "I administer skilled essential care that returns patients to optimum levels of function." Nor are you likely to hear, "I restore health and well-being, and I provide comfort and care for the elderly," or "I ease pain," or "I support rehabilitation," or "I assist the dying in making their transition," or any of the myriad of vital, indispensible services that nurses provide almost

as second nature. What many will say is task oriented—"I give meds," or "I provide wound care," or "I do everything someone else doesn't do," or "I do all the scut work," and so forth.

What is almost a given is that nurses will not quote either the International Council of Nurses (ICN) or the American Nurses Association (ANA) definition of nursing, which will be discussed further in the epilogue. It is so much jargon that is hard to read, a mouthful to say, and difficult to apply. Perhaps it is good for the classroom, but the classroom is not good enough for the practice environment. Neither is it good enough for nurses to explain to the public with any degree of confidence that they will be understood and respected for the vital role they play, and that is another reason I have written this book. Although in some parts of the country nurses are earning well, overall, nurses have not achieved the status or pay rates richly deserved—congruent with the important contribution nurses make to society. Further, I believe that simpler is better. Let us tell it like it is in language that is understood by the broadest segment of our own practitioners and to society.

This book addresses these essential factors and more. Although it is written from the bedside, it is strong on theory, with phenomenology being the overarching hypothesis. The framework is theoretically sound—praxis prevails.

A contribution is made by noted author and educator Patricia Munhall, EdD, RN, PsyA, FAAN, who explains the theoretical foundation of this book—phenomenology—in the prologue. Who better to enlighten the reader about what it is like to walk a mile in another's shoes than someone who is noted for her research and writings in this field?

Much of what I have written is from observation and interaction with patients, nurses, nurse managers, entry-level and interdisciplinary staff, colleagues, administrators, and physicians, friends and family members as well as from personal experience during my work life and educational and consulting experience. Nothing has been fabricated.

Because a large percentage of nursing still is comprised of women, I have used the pronoun *she* throughout the book. This in no way is meant to discount or disrespect the major and increasing contribution to nursing and to patient care made by our male counterparts. It is just that he/she or she/he is awkward and a mouthful if someone chooses to read *Patient-Centered Care . . .* aloud.

It is my sincere hope that readers will enjoy reading *Patient-Centered Care* and that it will become a source of information that can be applied to, and improve, practice.

Nursing—An Influential Profession

There is just one more thing I would like to say by way of introducing myself to you as you prepare to spend some time with me. What follows is my first foray into nursing. This is when the idea entered my mind and never left. It is why I decided to become a nurse in the first place.

When I was about 8 years old, I started reading the Cherry Ames nurse series of books. I found the stories exciting and motivational. I was already the kind of kid who liked to fix people and pets. Blood and gore did not repel me—they fascinated me. So my mother gave me an anatomy and physiology book with transparent overlays. Its medical aid section taught me a lot about stanching blood and disinfecting wounds. She hoped it would motivate me to become a doctor. But Cherry and nursing always won out over every other thing that came my way.

Ideas like, "The first duty of a nurse is always to her patient," struck my altruistic core; "spending extra time with sick and injured children and practicing holistic nursing" seemed the right thing to do—even though I had to look up the word holistic.

Cherry learned that part of holistic nursing included "psycho-neurological nursing," and so did I. When I discovered that Cherry had a "propensity for bending the rules," I felt a kinship with her. When I learned of her curiosity, intelligence, and courage, I aspired to be described in those terms. Finally, I learned that nursing was a profession of influential women—just like the family in which I had grown and developed.

At 17, I entered nursing school and have stayed with the profession ever since. Never have I regretted that choice. During the ensuing decades, I have seen examples of superb nursing care that has healed body, heart, and mind. I have observed nurses help patients replace fear with hope and assist individuals, families, and populations regain health and optimism they never thought possible.

But there are always two sides to every coin. As humanistic professionals, we deserve to rejoice in the excellent service we provide, in the wonderful work we do, in the superhuman effort we offer to those who come to us for care no matter their race, religion, national origin, or ability to pay. But we also must be willing to examine our failures as well. In truth, the only way we can define and perpetuate what is good is by knowing and understanding what is bad.

Nursing Leadership for Patient-Centered Care is a practical approach to fixing what is broken. It is not meant to denigrate or insult a quality profession essential to the health and welfare of individuals and the greater society—or its individual practitioners. To do that would be to denigrate myself. But to ignore breakdowns in care is to allow them to self-perpetuate. It also risks having patients endure substandard care and to dread facing institutional encounters.

Prologue

Listening With the Third Ear: Or—The Philosophical Underpinnings of This Book

Patricia Munhall, EdD, ARNP, PsyA, FAAN

In the beginner's mind, there are many possibilities, but in the expert's mind there are few. —**Suzuki Shunryu**

This Zen Master's quote introduces us to the paradoxical nature of everything we have been taught. Quotes such as this succinctly provide us some of the wisest ideas to ponder. People's narratives of their experiences in whatever context they may appear also offer us insights into their experiences—how they felt, how they were influenced, what it meant to *them*.

Today's popular literature is often replete with first-person narratives. Because they are "real," they hold readers in awe and provide them with pathways to understanding.

This book, *Nursing Leadership for Patient-Centered Care*, does just that. It offers the reader an opportunity to understand what is actually occurring in nursing leadership and management, as well as in nursing practice at the bedside.

Later in this prologue, I will discuss the philosophical perspective of phenomenology, which, in basic terms, attempts to understand the meaning of another person's experience. To understand others, though, you need a beginner's mind—a fun place to be, because of the many possibilities of understanding that open up to you. Some of these possibilities you might not have imagined before.

"The greatest obstacle to discovery is not ignorance but the illusion of knowledge." This quote by Daniel J. Boorstin, a prize-winning author and former librarian of congress, illustrates the notion that, if we think we know something, we do not look for answers. I call this premature closure to understanding an experience to its fullest, richest depth. A song by Tom Petty and the Heartbreakers also illustrates this point: "You don't know how it

1

feels to be me." I start each phenomenology workshop with this song. The chorus, repeated often, conveys in great clarity what phenomenology as a perspective attempts to resolve.

You might find this CD, entitled *Wildflowers*, worth the investment. Then, you can play it over and over again, so that you can begin to realize, even at a visceral level, how little we understand, really understand others. Often we say to someone, "I don't know why I did that or why I said that." In other words, we also struggle to understand ourselves.

There are many ways to approach the project of human understanding. But if we have been taught one way, adapted one theory, accepted it, applied it to staff or to patients, and it failed to work, then what?

We have to remember that each person we encounter can help us discover what is best for him or for her—if we remain open to learning. The other person, not us, is the expert on him or herself. Often, as nurse leaders and managers, or in patient care, we try to fit the staff or patient into *our* theory, when actually *that other person* should provide direction for a particular and individualizing theory; that is, once we understand that individual's interior (subjective) world.

Dr. Forman's book is about gaining that understanding from first-person narratives or stories: what happened to them, how it was for them, what they felt like, how they experienced the event, and importantly, what we should know about various sectors of the health care arena in this regard. How nurses and patients perceive conditions and procedures provides direction for nurse leaders and managers.

THIS IS THE HOW OF THIS BOOK

This book shows those in nursing leadership and management how to understand what is occurring on the units and at the bedside by listening to the people involved: the patient, the patient's family, the staff nurse, the nurse manager, physicians, or members of support services departments such as housekeepers and transporters, among others. They tell us what is going on through their own perceptions of various situations. This produces *authentic-based knowledge*. Evidence-based practice, of course, has its place. But caution, here, also has its place when implementing such practice within general protocols—which are developed for the "average" person who might not exist, in fact. Best is to get to know each person as a *unique individual*. You might remember that concept from your first nursing class.

Dr. Forman, in writing this book, reflects the narratives of many different individuals. As you read their stories, you realize the need to understand and know them from the perspective of their uniqueness. Nurse leaders and managers are asked to put aside preconceptions so they can discover the many areas that are begging for their expertise and intervention. The best place to start is always by listening to those who are living, or who have lived, through the experience.

Nurse leaders and managers have a high calling. They navigate a challenging workplace with limited resources, conflicts to solve, complaints to resolve, patient complications, and patient care errors to prevent or to correct. It is a calling that requires courage and direction. This book provides a pathway lit by the voices of patients and family members, of nurses and other personnel.

ANOTHER HOW OF THIS BOOK: PHILOSOPHICAL CONCEPTUAL ANALYSIS

We gain insight into what constitutes the best nursing management/leadership practice, in general, by talking about imperfect scenarios, along with good scenarios. This is a *philosophical* process of conceptual analysis (different from the one we use in nursing). In this process, we first ask the question: "What is good nursing management?" (Soltis, 1968). Then, according to this process, we identify two categories as exemplars. In one category, we note those characteristics of excellent nursing management using examples to illustrate each point. In the other category, we note the characteristics of imperfect nursing management. The idea is that, to know what is good, we must also and always look critically at what might be considered poor nursing management.

UNDERSTANDING THE OTHER: THE THIRD EAR

Think of all the misunderstandings you experience in just one day, and all the chaos this causes. For the patient, misunderstanding can generate frustration, powerlessness, miscommunication, feelings of isolation, or even oppression. The complications often include medical and nursing errors such as pressure injuries, contractures, infections, and even death.

How about misunderstanding among staff? Think about the disastrous implications from labeling and gossiping, criticism, poor coordination and delivery of care, and arguments. Some of the worst outcomes may be work place mobbing (Duffy, 2009) or work place violence, whether psychological or physical.

What is critical, in order to understand another person, is to suspend our assumptions, presuppositions, and even our book knowledge. We need to listen with what has been called the "third ear." This requires an open mind that embraces discovery and welcomes possibilities. To do this, we must temporarily set aside what we think or know and listen carefully.

Not only should the patient be heard with this "third ear," but also everyone else on the health care team. The modeling of this listening and the teaching of "how" to listen with the third ear is part of being the outstanding nurse manager.

HOLISTIC PRACTICE INVOLVES MORE THAN THE PATIENT

This brings me to the people we encounter each day in the workplace—the nurse leaders and managers who often feel overwhelmed. Are we going to add the dimension of understanding the staff as a holistic group of individuals, from the housekeeper to the attending physician, to their already over-the-top responsibilities?

The answer is yes, because it will promote the concept that they all deserve equal treatment as human beings, because it is the just and ethical way to practice, and because it will lead to greater success in a leadership role. Rather than extra work, it will eliminate the fallout, as mentioned above, that comes from "not understanding" and from miscommunication.

Rather then making life more difficult for the nurse in a leadership role, the time spent in understanding others and their experiences will make life less stressful, more successful, and as an added benefit, more rewarding. Taking time to understand the context and contingencies of another person's life *in the moment* individualizes that person's uniqueness.

LEAVE YOUR TROUBLES ON THE DOORSTEP

This idea of not taking "stuff" to work is naïve. Once we are on a unit, we cannot leave behind emotionally laden issues such as a dying mother, a sick child, a home in foreclosure, or a failing marriage.

Practicing nursing management from this holistic perspective is guaranteed to improve workplace morale, camaraderie, and cooperation. It ensures better nursing care. These are the benefits of taking the time and interest to listen. In contrast (remember conceptual analysis), perhaps the nurse manager is humanistic toward patients, but not particularly with her staff. Until she abdicates her "knowing" position—the position of power, assumptions, and expectations without considering the context of the staff member's life in the moment—she will unfortunately be practicing a very mechanistic form of management.

Often, the prescription for this type of nursing management comes from textbooks. These prescriptions may be formulaic, given without context or contingency considerations. They have their place in that they provide a framework. But that framework must then be individualized.

A few last thoughts which I think are critical: This cannot be faked. It must be authentic. Being a nurse leader or manager is a position of privilege as opposed to power. One of the best characteristics of a nurse leader/manager is being attuned to the staff's lives, and to understand them as individuals. If you do not believe me, ask a staff nurse if she or he agrees. Ask the nurse aide.

Too often staff members feel dehumanized. Remember "horizontal violence" (Roberts, 1983), which Dr. Forman covers later in this book. Briefly, not being able to address others in power, the staff practices destructive behavior to one another. Nurse managers who listen to the narratives of their staff in demonstrable ways, and show they are actually paying attention, eliminate many of these energy-depleting scenarios.

NOW TO THE CRUX OF THE MATTER: UNDERSTANDING ANOTHER IN AN EXPERIENCE

Before beginning a more detailed analysis of understanding the other, whether staff member or patient, I hope I have convinced you that this is not "more to do," "impractical," or "too soft," but actually the path to becoming a successful nurse leader/manager. Some of what I am about to present may be familiar to those who have taken research courses and, in particular, have learned about qualitative research. No worries, though, even if you have not studied this, because I am not going to present the approach from the research perspective. I will present it as a way that is exemplified in this book: *how to listen, how to understand another,* and *how to identify with the experience of others.* This will be essentially a description of the method Dr. Forman has used in this book—a page turner you will enjoy reading, and from which you will learn in a way you might find unfamiliar.

To discover what is necessary to understand the other, let us start with a quote from Thomas Henry Huxley, a nineteenth century English biologist. He said,

> Sit down before the fact like a little child, and be prepared to give up every preconceived notion, following humbly wherever and to whatever abyss nature leads or you shall learn nothing.

To understand another and even yourself, it is essential to acknowledge your preconceptions, beliefs, intuitions, motives, biases, and knowledge base. Remain open to a whole new perception of another or yourself. This is also a critical component of the philosophical *phenomenological* perspective that I try to live by.

This is the guiding framework for this book.

THE PHENOMENOLOGICAL PERSPECTIVE: THE SUBJECTIVE STUDY OF EXPERIENCE

I am glad to say—since many of us have invested much of our professional lives in advancing this way of thinking—that many nurses have come to embrace it. Those who are hesitant comprise a more scientific, fact-seeking, quantitatively oriented group, and they are needed. This is not a conversion-seeking discussion. The phenomenological perspective is a philosophy that seeks to understand the meaning of experiences for other people. The goal is to understand how individuals are experiencing what they are confronting.

As nurses, we see people when they are at their most vulnerable, at risk, in fragile conditions. It is critical that we find out what is going on inside them. What is it that they are experiencing? Is it anxiety, powerlessness, loss of self, fear of dying, pain, hopelessness, loneliness, and all the myriad of unique responses people have to illness and their experience of illness? From these perceptions, we plan nursing care. This is based on understanding the patient and his or her needs. There are no textbooks or protocols that can predict how an individual will interpret his experience or reality. This is where we need to listen with the "third ear." This is how the nurse leader/manager meets her responsibilities to both patients and staff.

As a nurse leader and manager who has the potential to create an environment of caring, compassion, and also the most excellent nursing care delivered, the same dynamic applies. She or he needs to understand the experience of all the members of the health care team. What meanings are they giving to what they perceive and to what they actually experience? Are they afraid and feeling inadequate, stressed, dealing with personal trauma, and perhaps distracted, or overwhelmed? Are they angry about their working conditions? Are they feeling tension and competition among staff? Do they feel that the nurse manager has favorites, or conversely, do they feel appreciated and respected?

Can you see how responses to experiences can be different for each person, patient, or staff member? Considering the variety of these responses, think how impossible it would be to have a one-way-fits-all model, which as mentioned, can lead to miscommunication, misunderstanding, and medical and nursing errors.

This book attests to the variety of circumstances that can occur, how individuals respond, and how—too often—practice is jeopardized. Where did the perception start that being in a hospital is dangerous?

If nurse managers and staff turned their attention to the subjective worlds of staff and patients, we could hopefully turn that perception around. This is a task of no small consequence, I admit. However, if we were to learn more about what is perceived as alarming, as this book clearly articulates, then an essential new paradigm for care would emerge.

In the *New York Times* Science Section (12/7/09), there was an article stating a frightening fact—more than half of the patients in intensive care units have infections, and they are more than twice as likely to die in the units as those who are infection free. These patients are in intensive care units for life-threatening conditions, but they do not die from those conditions. They die from what we call iatrogenesis, hospital-acquired conditions. Since objective knowledge has its limits in solving this problem, perhaps we need to look at the subjective worlds of all concerned.

This article refers to mostly respiratory infections, and hand washing is mentioned. In her book, Dr. Forman refers to a case in which a patient in an ICU suffers a stage-V infected pressure ulcer while on one-on-one care in an ICU. His nurse attributes this to diarrhea.

The question arises: what is the subjective world, or the interior world experience of a staff member who perhaps "cuts corners" in a particular situation? Is a demoralized staff member more likely to do this? To find out, we need to examine and understand each person's phenomenological perspective.

HOW DO WE PRACTICE (OR WRITE) FROM THE PHENOMENOLOGICAL PERSPECTIVE?

Vignette   Phenomenology—A Funny-Sounding Word

While I was working on my doctoral dissertation concerning phenomenology, my was in third grade. As with many children his age, he seemed to like funny-sounding words. Hearing me often repeat the word phenomenology, he readily picked up and used this "wordy" word. After listening to my explanation, he thought it meant to situate oneself in the place of the "other" to understand that other person. So in an essay he was writing on bullying, he inserted the word phenomenology as a way to combat bullying.

Of course this scored some points with his teacher, who called me to ask what the word phenomenology meant. Once I explained it to her, she agreed. Subsequently, she taught her students to imagine how it "feels" to be bullied—the sentiment expressed in the Tom Petty song. From a phenomenological perspective, though, we would go one step further and ask some children who had been bullied to describe the experience in their own words and the meanings they attached to these unfortunate experiences.

While you are reading this book, you are actually reading the phenomenological perspectives of nurse leaders, nurse managers, staff, family members, and patients. Therefore, you have examples of how revealing it is to hear people describe their experiences. These are rich narratives that will provide direction for practice.

You might ask, "Isn't that the same as empathy?" Empathy is often described as putting oneself in others' shoes and *feeling* as they feel.

We do that with phenomenology in a way, but instead—and this is a big *INSTEAD*—we do not assume that we know the pain and suffering of others—that our feelings are the same as are their feelings or that we perceive experience in a similar manner. Instead, we *ask them* to talk to us from their own experience. As mentioned previously, we honor their uniqueness and all the possibilities of their individual responses and feelings. We want to know how *they* are experiencing something but also what meaning it has for them. If we were to limit our understanding of others to our own perspectives, then we would be coming from our own interior world. It would be about us and our subjective stance toward the world. It would rely on our own beliefs, values, perceptions, and knowledge—all the components mentioned earlier that need to be suspended when approaching an experience phenomenologically. We do not interpret the experience for another. We encourage the individual to have the freedom to interpret his or her own experience. This is what you will be doing when you read the narratives and stories told in this book. You will have the authentic account, not one you interpreted from your own life experiences.

This is critical. The sequence of events that opens this book and the one in the epilogue are examples of phenomenological narratives. They are first-person accounts with all the attendant feelings, responses, and meanings articulated from the persons who *experienced* the phenomenon.

So you can see where the term *phenomenology* comes from. Philosophy, like most disciplines, has its own vocabulary. Instead of simply calling a situation an experience, philosophers called it a phenomenon. Technically, with "ology" added, phenomenology is the study of phenomena. But it could just as easily be called the study of experience.

THE ROAD TO UNDERSTANDING: THE INTERSUBJECTIVENESS OF "WE-NESS"

I hope that the argument for the importance of understanding the uniqueness of another, and her or his perception of an experience, has been understood. Recall that the way the nurse leader/manager can best perform her role is to understand the holistic nature of all who are in her environment. She needs to appreciate how people experience and attach meaning to being on the staff in order to produce the best results in the most humanistic, compassionate, and effective ways possible.

How patients and staff view their reality, what they are experiencing and feeling, what meaning *they* attach needs to be understood by all concerned. Everyone is intertwined. There is a "we-ness" of two subjective worlds coming together creating an intersubjective space where understanding becomes possible (further discussed in next section). By assuming a phenomenological perspective, the nurse leader/manger ensures that the staff and patient experience is understood; she provides compassion and understanding that is individualized for staff and patients alike. This improves patient outcomes and decreases complications and errors. That it also makes the work experience gratifying is another one of its greatest rewards.

AUTHENTIC LISTENING—HOW AND WHAT

Now down to the "how" of authentic listening, in order to understand, without "the illusion of knowledge." Let me explain how I am using the word "perception" for the purposes of this prologue and also how it is structured as the framework for this book. First a question: which comes first—subjectivity or perception? The answer is that both are essential to the existence of the other. They are simultaneous in nature. But first, one must perceive.

Perception

Perception is largely how we *individually* view the world and all its parts and regarding this book, how we view the role of the nurse leader/manager and the all-inclusive staff.

Throughout the course of our own personal development, we appropriate various beliefs, values, intuitions, preconceptions, assumptions, book knowledge, and inherited knowledge from others. This includes biases and everything else that adds up to our worldview, from the topic of this book to the color blue. Perceptions that are built on prejudices and partiality (addressed in this book) can be extremely harmful. When we attempt to understand another individual, everything that contributes to our perceptions—especially prejudices and predispositions—should all be held in abeyance. That is, to the extent possible for us, we must disregard and place aside anything that has contributed to our own perception of something. This step is absolutely essential to obtain a true understanding of another person.

It is in the common parlance that our perceptions create our own reality. We all have different perceptions of the same reality. This is a cause for conflict and disagreements as we are often talking right past a person. A self-help book that you might have read demonstrates this vividly. It is John Gray's, *Men are from Mars, Women are from Venus* (1992). This book illustrates in a fun and informative way why men and women are so often in conflict. Each sees reality from what Gray tells us is from two completely different sets of perceptions. If you have not read the book, I strongly recommend it to improve your relationships with the opposite sex—in both the personal and professional realm.

In addition, "what WE would do" in that person's situation, also must be placed aside. What might be good for one person may be inappropriate or even disastrous for another.

So, in phenomenological understanding, the *knower* is the person whom we are trying to understand. We should not question the validity of the knower. Whatever that person reports is that person's perception. Whether we agree or disagree, our aim is to understand how that individual is viewing an experience. Our opinion should not be running along parallel to the person talking to us.

I have used the following technique and admit it takes practice. Simply, I keep my mouth shut or use words to encourage the person to continue. I have heard and probably have been guilty as well of statements like, "but don't you think" or, "that is not really what is happening." But you can see how that would interfere with understanding the authentic telling of the person's experience. So when you read Dr. Forman's book, you might hear yourself saying, "but that could not be helped" or "that is exaggerated". I urge you to suspend interjecting your own perceptions at the moment of reading. Let each example in this book have his or her own voice, his or her own telling of the experience, his or her own perceptions of the event.

Intersubjectivity

Each of us has our own subjective worldview, our own window to interpreting the world and all that it holds. Residing in our subjective world, or the subjective part of our consciousness, are our perceptions. The other part of our consciousness is sometimes referred to as an objective world. We might interpret that objectivity as *agreed upon facts*.

Philosophers have argued about objectivity, or lack of it, for eons. Objective facts are supposedly immutable—unchangeable—so we do not have to argue about them like we might about our subjective world. But we all have an idea as to how many so-called objective facts have not held up through time. So it is a good idea to be cautious with "facts."

We are sometimes told to be objective or to give an objective opinion. From my perspective, these two ideas are going to wind up being subjective. I recall hearing at a conference once, that *objectivity is a subjective notion*. That works for me, but not for everyone. Also, it is another chapter for another book!

We are speaking about *inter*subjectivity. What this means is when two or more people come together, there is a melding of the different subjectivities.

Therefore, when we are conversing, each person speaks from her or his own subjective world with individual respective perceptions. An intersubjective space then opens up with this mergence of two subjectivities. In this space, as mentioned, filled with individual perceptions, conflicts, disagreements, and agreements take place. So it is a place worthy of our critical attention.

WHAT MAKES IT PHENOMENOLOGICAL IS TO OBTAIN UNDERSTANDING OF THE OTHER

Now that we have arrived at this point, I once again encourage you to read Dr. Forman's book from this phenomenological perspective, especially since it was written that way.

GIVE VOICE TO ANOTHER WITHOUT YOUR OWN OVERLAP

This means, in this instance and with individuals you are attempting to understand, that you acknowledge your subjective consciousness. Hold your perceptions in abeyance. Place your subjectivity on the shelf and listen without the noise of self—listen with your third ear.

This is the phenomenological idea of the use of intersubjectivity in the *pursuit* of understanding the experience of another and for *understanding* that experience. As to the intersubjective space: you remove your own subjective stance and allow the other to eclipse yours. Then, you will be able to hear how that person actually experiences a phenomenon in the most authentic way.

IN THIS BOOK AND IN YOUR EXPERIENCE

An excellent place to start "listening" with your third ear is right here, with this book. Some of you may object to depictions of experiences by the narrator, patients, or staff. That is your subjective response. However, if you were to listen in an intersubjective way, you would suspend your subjective response and read the narrative or example as presented—it is a true telling of an experience from another person's subjective world. *That world as told in the narrative is authentic for that person.* Hearing it and accepting it, even if at first it might offend, offers great opportunity for professional and personal growth.

WANTED: NURSE MANAGERS WHO LISTEN WITH THE THIRD EAR

We need excellent nurse leaders, managers, and nurses who are able to listen with the third ear to staff, patients, and families. They should be in a holistic environment where they feel welcomed to talk without prejudice or fear, where they welcome the other's subjective experience, where they are completely respectful of other's subjective world. The nurse leader/manager realizes this is the person's authentic perception of the experience. This nurse leader/manager is rewarded by a rich and satisfying practice.

Listening to another person's interpretation of their experiences—and responding with thoughtfulness, respect, kindness, compassion, generosity, caring, and authenticity—is the path to individualized leadership and management practice, as well as excellent nursing care. Using the phenomenological perspective to listen keeps the noise out, so that staff and patient voices are heard with clarity like the ring of fine crystal. The nurse leader/manager has a special calling; she is a unique individual who can create change so that another book like this may not be needed. That is my desire for all nurse managers, nurses, auxiliary staff, patients, and their families. Utopian thinking? Perhaps, but it gives us all a goal.

In her epilogue, Dr. Forman refers to a quote from the Kaballah about the end being in its beginning. I would like to follow suit. Since I began with a quote about possibilities, I would like to end with one as well, one that illustrates what nurses need to acknowledge about all those individuals in their environment, including themselves. This one is from Peter Senge who said, "We need to be the authors of our own life."

CHAPTER ENDNOTES

Duffy, M. 2009. Preventing workplace mobbing and bullying with effective organizational consultation, policies and legislation. *Consulting Psychology Journal: Practice and Research* 61(3):242–262.

Huxley, J. H. 1982. In: L. Dossey, *Time, space and medicine*. Colorado: Shambhala.

Roberts, S. J. 1983. Oppressed group behavior: Implications for nursing. *Advances in Nursing Science* 5:21–30.

Soltis, J. 1968. *An introduction to the analysis of educational concepts*. Reading, MA: Addison-Wesley.

1

The Three Cs: Collaboration, Communication, and Cooperation

Coming together is a beginning. Keeping together is progress. Working together is success. —*Henry Ford*

NURSE/PATIENT COLLABORATION, COMMUNICATION, AND COOPERATION

Vignette   Setting the Stage With a Merkel Cell Carcinoma

A Merkel cell carcinoma—a rare aggressive type of skin cancer—had been surgically excised from the patient's upper thigh by a well-reputed surgeon in a renowned medical center. Ten days later, as the sutures were being removed, the wound dehisced and bled profusely. The surgeon packed the wound, which measured 15×8 cm, and was 5 cm deep, and released the patient with a referral to a home nursing service.

The next morning, a nurse arrived, assessed the wound, and told the patient that he needed to be in the hospital. She then contacted the surgeon to make the necessary arrangements.

The patient and his wife packed a bag and headed for the admissions department to complete the paper work. The clerk directed them to the specified floor and unit.

By the time they arrived, the patient was exhausted, and they could not find his room. There were no clear signs, and no one was in sight to ask. Finally, they located the room—a double with two unmade beds. Linen was piled on an air exchange unit. Neither bed was occupied nor had they any idea to which bed he had been assigned. They claimed the bed near the window and the wife settled her husband into a chair. She pressed the nurse call button. No one responded.

After 10 minutes, the wife made the bed and helped her husband to lie down. She noticed blood soaking through his trousers.

Alarmed, she located a nurse and told her about it. The nurse said she could do nothing without a doctor's orders and walked away.

The patient's wife rifled through drawers and closets until she found gauze and tape with which she reinforced the dressing. Then she went to the desk and found a resident physician who said he could come in 7 minutes, but not immediately.

This was the beginning of a week of care that was anything but patient-centered. That is what this book is about: patient-centered care that is all too often lacking in today's beleaguered health care system. It is also about health care professionals and support staff who appear exhausted, have unclear missions and goals, and seem to suffer from ambiguous leadership and uncertain management. They are battling a myriad of these and other self-defeating issues that thwart even the most motivated professionals.

The nurse, in the above scenario, was wrong when she said she needed a doctor's order to treat the bleeding wound. Her responsibility at the time was to that patient. In a patient-centered environment, she would have known that. This is the very definition of nursing under the American Nurses Association's (ANA) Social Policy Statement. In fact, her hospital had achieved Magnet Status (ANA: Nursing Administration Scope & Standards of Practice, 2009)—and had she understood what that meant, she would have known that her organization was expected to deliver excellent patient outcomes.

Had the nurse studied Nightingale or Henderson, founders of modern nursing, she would have known that the nurse is responsible for doing for the patient that which the patient would do for himself—had he the capacity to do so. Sadly, by her actions, she seemed to be unaware of any of these things—only that she could turn her back and walk away.

During the entire week of hospitalization, not one nurse discussed the patient's diagnosis or possible outcomes with him. They gave him his meds and dressed his wound per MD's orders. They attended to the tasks.

He had a grievous wound and was seen by a dietician who recommended a high-protein diet. She advised his wife to bring at least one such meal each day from home because it was unlikely that the hospital meals would meet his protein needs.

Because there was a contaminant in the water system, he could not use the bathroom shower or sink. No one offered to assist him with the packaged bed bath that was supplied to him with the linen. He had to ask.

Here is another story of lack of cooperation, collaboration, and communication between a patient and members of a nursing service that resulted in unacceptable care. In this case, the patient signed herself out of a hospital against medical advice (AMA), thus jeopardizing her health and ultimately the hospital's malpractice standing.

Vignette **From the Mouth of the Patient**

Having had several bouts of viral meningitis, when I had familiar symptoms I went to the emergency room of my hospital. By the time I got there I was in excruciating pain. The ER was packed. I was put on a stretcher and left in the hallway among other patients for nearly ten hours covered only with my jacket. Finally, a staff member rolled my stretcher into an isolation room. There I was told by a nurse that there were no blankets or pillows available. There was neither a bathroom in the isolation room nor a commode. After several unattended hours I needed to void and called out for help. No one responded. I got off the stretcher. Weak and in excruciating pain I stood at the door and called out. Still no one responded. I walked out of the isolation room and fainted.

Just then, the patient's parents arrived and as they later described it, they were shaken by the flurry of activity surrounding their daughter. They later learned that she had not been given even a sheet or blanket despite the well-stocked linen carts they had seen near the ER entrance. Also, they were distressed to learn that a bedside commode had not been supplied, that the many calls to the staff had been ignored, and that their daughter's pain had not been addressed. There had been no collaboration between the nursing staff and this patient who had been left without essential care for many hours.

This too, was a Magnet Hospital. Nevertheless, nursing was unavailable to this patient, and according to the parents, to the many patients who lay on stretchers in the corridor separating the glass-enclosed centralized nursing station from the examining rooms. Each patient's privacy was minimally protected by a portable screen. Instead of sheets or blankets, they were covered only by their coats and jackets.

Eventually, this patient was transferred, first to a temporary room assignment to clear ER space and then to her room. As the patient continues:

I was there for less than an hour when an orderly entered the room with a wheelchair to transfer me to another room. I told him that I would need a gurney since I could not sit up. He came back with one and told me to get on it. I told him I needed assistance—a step stool or something. He got one but offered no help. As he was wheeling me out of the room he coughed without covering his nose and mouth. Several days later—because of lack of attention and poor care—I decided to check out AMA. The night before discharge, I called the nurse and told her that I was very cold and was shivering uncontrollably. She told me I was having an anxiety attack about going home the next day, and that I should sleep. I awoke in the middle of the night feeling as if my lungs and throat were on fire. I pressed the call button for about 10 minutes, but nobody responded. Finally I went to the main desk and demanded that someone take my temperature. They begrudgingly complied until they saw that my temperature was 106°F. They packed me in ice and gave me Tylenol. I left the next morning—against medical advice—believing myself in danger due to poor care.

Discussion: The parents wrote to the chief nurse executive (CNE) and received a pro forma response. As you read this and the other vignettes in this chapter, think about how these situations might have been better handled, bearing in mind that short staffing is a reality in health care today and is likely to worsen. Also, consider that most of the hospitals I am discussing have well-educated individuals at the helm—at least masters prepared. At the upper leadership levels, some have earned doctorates. All facilities are Joint Commission accredited and many have been awarded Magnet Status. The vignettes described here, reported by patients, their significant others, and the author and other professionals including nurses, physicians, and therapists among others, should be carefully considered. Questions about what went wrong and what could have been done to offer better, more professional, more satisfying care, need to be answered.

STAFF: MANAGEMENT/LEADERSHIP COLLABORATION, COMMUNICATION, COOPERATION

The previous story was from the patient's perspective and took place in suburban New York. Here is another story about lack of collaboration, communication, and cooperation, this time between staff and leadership. It happened in a large voluntary hospital in the south where staff members felt they were not valued by management.

The CEO of a 570-bed acute care hospital conducted monthly staff meetings in the auditorium. All available staff members, from the groundskeepers to the administrators, were invited to attend and "speak their minds." Many took part even though, based on past history, follow-through seemed unlikely. One day, a staff RN, known to share his views freely, was about to enter the auditorium. His supervisor, with a snide smile on her face approached him and lifted his ID badge. "Remember," she said "I know who you are." The RN took this to mean "keep your mouth shut!"

Soon after the meeting ended, word of this incident spread like wildfire. The supervisor said she had just been kidding. Had her staff trusted her, they might have believed her. But based on her past behavior, which was punitive and authoritarian, that was not the case; therefore, it was too late to stop the negative cascade that her words started.

Groups of staff members gathered in corners and discussed the event. Like the children's game of telephone, with each repetition, the version changed. Instead of the supervisor having said, "I know who you are," by the end of the week, the message became, "if you open your mouth and say one word, I'll fire you."

Nothing management could say or do seemed able to put out the rapidly spreading conflagration. Confidence was low. Communication flowed in one direction: from top down. Managers had not established one-on-one relationships with individual staff members, so there was little or no communication from the bottom up. Also, patient-focused language was not the norm. Me's, you's, and we's were standard, and this caused competition instead of cooperation. Staff members talked about contacting unions to represent them against management. Things were going from bad to worse.

Finally, the CNE called in a consultant to see what he could do to break the stalemate that had hardened the staff. He asked for a meeting with the most outspoken, angry, and obdurate nurses to see if they would participate in a focus group. Many stepped forward; 20 were chosen by lottery.

At the start of the meeting, he announced that they were welcome to contribute anonymously. To a person, they declined to remove their ID badges. Attendance was not taken.

It was an open forum. The nurses painted a picture of poor leadership and management. Examples started with the monthly CEO meetings, after which there was seldom any follow-up. The CEO's agenda was task and physical plant, not staff or patient oriented. He listened, but that is where it ended. He neither promised nor provided solutions to the problems the staff articulated. This in itself was demotivating.

Supervisors, like the one who started the problem, were archetypal. Managers did not work at establishing relationships with staff members; they were mostly absent from their units, and when they were there, they clung to their clipboards and rarely lent a hand. They tended to be authoritative, punitive, and demanding. Instead of supporting staff, they placed blame—often in front of patients and others. Also, they played favorites, ensuring that their friends received preferential scheduling, performance appraisals, and promotions.

By the time the meeting's allotted hour ended, the consultant had six legal-size pages of notes—grievances actually—against management. They asked the consultant what he intended to do. He replied that he would report back to the CNE who had invited him in with his recommendations for an action plan that would include periodic meetings with this same group to review their perception of progress.

The CNE, who was relatively new to the organization, practiced MBWA. She was a warm person who was humanistic by nature, and expressed concern for both patients and staff. Regular three-shift rounds and around-the-clock staff meetings were routine for her, and she arranged with the consultant to conduct professional management seminars and leadership workshops. Next, she arranged for substandard managers to be counseled, participate in remediation, and if unable to rise to new standards, let go and replaced.

As promised, the consultant met regularly with the original group that had become the steering committee and the voice of the staff. They reported an improvement in morale, which took a bounce when the punitive supervisor—the one who started the furor in the first place—was replaced with a patient- and staff-oriented professional manager.

The staff noticed steady improvements in communication, leadership skills, management visibility, and interaction on the units. Monthly administrative meetings continued, and there was follow-up on issues raised. Staff members were beginning to believe that management cared about them as individuals and hope started to replace anger. They now could turn their attention to their patients. The new formula in which management cares for staff, in turn, motivating staff to care for patients, was starting to take root.

On a return visit—one to gauge leadership style and effectiveness—the consultant asked the steering committee about leadership styles.

He wanted to know if staff members:

▪ Felt safe to disagree without fear of reprisal.

▪ Were included in decision making.

▪ Were *not* spoken down to or felt demeaned.

▪ Were praised publically and criticized privately.

▪ Had opportunities for promotion based on demonstrated expertise.

▪ Had opportunities to present new ideas that would improve patient outcome and ease their workload.

▪ Believed they were working with patient-centered leaders who demonstrated positive behavioral styles and communicated effectively.

▪ Cooperated and collaborated in a way that had a positive impact on patient care.

▪ Felt good working in that leadership environment and believed patients
felt good about the care they received.

▪ Experienced their managers as good role models and mentors.

The consensus opinion was that there was discernible improvement but
that insufficient time had transpired for trust to have replaced the former
levels of doubt. The phrase "time will tell" seemed to be their position.

At this point, a word or two about the concepts of *demonstrated expertise* versus *years of experience* used as a parameter for employment and
advancement. I have observed individuals with decades of work experience
whose skill sets did not compare favorably to relative neophytes who aced
everything they took on. Yet I continue to see—in recruitment ads and ads
for management and leadership advancement—a requirement for "at least
five years of experience." Also, there is a tendency in nursing to be narrow-
minded about educational requirements for leadership and academic positions. While in many other professions the doctorate rules, in nursing, even
for nonclinical positions, the master's degree often trumps the doctorate.
Employers frequently miss opportunities to mentor neophyte nurses and
enhance patient-centered care. I encourage readers to rethink their own
experience and how it translates to on-the-job expertise. The future rests
with you. Holding on to old habits and tired practice ensures a continuation
of old paradigms.

NURSING TEAM MEMBERS' COLLABORATION, COMMUNICATION, COOPERATION

The patient was comatose—obtunded. He also was overweight and required
several sets of staff member's hands to reposition him. With proper body

mechanics, two or three experienced nursing personnel could do it. Some insisted on a fourth.

Often, RNs entered the room and asked the family members where the NAs were. The family could always locate an aide or two, or more. The question was: why could the nurses not do so as well?

Upon investigation, it was learned that many of the nurses talked down to the NAs, and in so doing, diminished their worth, angered them, and made them want to get even. So they did, by making themselves unavailable to help out when needed. The conflict trickled down to the patients and resulted in a work environment that was not patient-centered. Support staff was uncooperative. Patients had to wait for care. This annoyed the RNs, and a vicious cycle was established.

The family members, on the other hand, valued the input of the NAs and showed their appreciation. All it took was a please, a thank you, and a how ya' doing?

There were other examples of RN misbehavior. For example, a medical student requested help from a nurse because he was having trouble drawing blood from a central line. Instead of offering immediate assistance, she made him wait. She had "other obligations," she said. These turned out to be powdering her nose, making a personal phone call, having a tête-à-tête with a colleague, and applying lipstick. Then, she returned to the bedside and assisted the beleaguered med student.

This patient's length of stay (LOS) was approximately 28 days, a long time in an acute care hospital. Although there was a nurse manager's office on the unit, the nurse manager never visited the patient. To make matters worse, there was a different *primary* nurse each day. When the family asked why, they were told that every nurse wanted to get to know every patient. This author has heard from a number of family members that "primary nurses" were changed daily during inpatient stays in a number of acute care hospitals in several large metropolitan areas. Although these individuals knew nothing about the theoretical framework behind primary nursing, they reported feeling disconcerted by frequent changes in staff.

In a third example from the same unit, the patient was returning from the OR on a special bed. The room he was assigned had a bed in it. The mother advised the unit clerk and suggested that the bed be removed so that her son need not wait in the hall. Several orderlies were standing by and could easily have handled it.

That would have been patient-centered behavior. Instead, the clerk, never looking up from her paper work, mumbled: "The transporters will take care of it."

Who Is at the Center of Attention in Patient-Centered Care?

There is no question that the patient's and his family's needs should have been the center of attention—not the nurses. But where was the nurse manager to oversee, mentor, and evaluate her staff in this philosophy? The family asked if she was off duty, but she was not. The nurses identified themselves as primary nurses, yet they ignored the philosophy of primary nursing.

To make matters worse, there were several patient care breakdowns. A Foley catheter was found by a family member to have been left clamped; the urine that had accumulated in the collection bag was scant and concentrated; an IV had "run out," and an air mattress had deflated. The nurses became defensive when informed.

Here are some questions to ponder when thinking about how these stories apply to your own practice:

- How would you have gone about shifting from these staff-centered philosophies and practices to patient-centered care?
- How would you find out if fear of reprisal was pervasive among patients and/or family members who complained about lack of consistency or nursing care breakdowns on this unit?
- What would you do about adversarial relationships between NAs and RNs?
- Define the steps you would take and the management/leadership support you would need.

This vignette speaks to the problem of patient care breakdowns and support staff not cooperating with professional licensed nurses. It spotlights the consequences of changing primary nurses daily because "they all want to get to know" patients on their unit. But this is clearly not patient-centered behavior.

What steps, if any, should the family have taken? In this case, the family provided care with some support from staff. Families and patients are often loathe to complain for fear of reprisal or "of making it worse." This is especially disturbing in cases where NAs roughly handle frail elderly patients. Adult children are often afraid to "make waves." Sometimes even racial or religious conflict is brought up as a concern.

One solution is for the nurse manager to be out and about on the units, among patients and staff. It does not take long for a skilled eye to see rough treatment or the *results* of rough treatment. Unfortunately, two things often interfere with taking action. One is short staffing, and the other is fear of retaliation or fear of a union. Neither of these are excuses.

Ask yourself these questions, and be painfully honest:

- How would you feel as a NA on that unit? Those NAs were angry and wanted to get back at the RNs. But disempowered, they simply made themselves unavailable.
- Do you consider support staff equal to you in all things other than professional licensure and all responsibilities that flow from that?
- Now, consider how and if you greet and treat your support team members—including the housekeeper who mops the floor.
- Given the opportunity, how would you go about shifting from egocentric behaviors to staff-centered/patient-centered care?

Here is a suggestion: start by asking patients how it *feels* to be cared for on your unit. Then do the same with your support staff. When you meet with them, really listen. Walk a mile in their shoes. Be empathetic. Feel their pain. Remember, empathy does not take time. It is an attitude, not a task.

One of the things that motivated me to write this book was a conversation I overheard on a New York City bus between two elderly women. One said to the other:

"I never want to have that experience again."

"What experience?" asked her companion.

"Having to be a patient in a hospital," answered the first woman.

"What happened?" queried the friend.

"I never felt so neglected, so vulnerable, so alone and uncared for in my life." the former patient said.

"My goodness," said her friend. "Where were you?"

The hospital named was a major, well-known medical center, Joint Commission accredited, affiliated with a medical school, and honored with Magnet Status. Still, the two elderly patients on that bus did not think much of its nursing care.

I went home and started to write a proposal to my publisher. For years, I had been thinking about writing a book of this kind and had been collecting vignettes. The one on the bus was my tipping point.

ROLES OF MANAGEMENT

An important role of management is to evaluate and improve staff effectiveness within and among the various disciplines. MBWA provides simultaneous observation of staff demeanor and behavior, staff interaction, and patient care intervention and outcomes. It also affords the manager opportunities to interact with patients and physicians, and to work alongside staff and mentor them in their clinical, observational, and communication skills.

In order for this to be effective, high levels of trust among and between staff and management must exist and endure. In the following vignette, trust was eroded. What follows is an account of revelation, evaluation, deconstruction, and reconstruction of an interdisciplinary team.

INTERDISCIPLINARY TEAM COLLABORATION, COMMUNICATION, AND COOPERATION

She was a consultant in a 300-bed suburban medical center that was part of a large horizontal health care system. Her charge was to work with middle management nursing staff to improve their leadership, management, and communication skills. Team building within the nursing department was to be closely followed by interdisciplinary cooperation and collaboration and improved labor relations. The ultimate goal was patient-centered care excellence.

One day, while making rounds on a medical unit, a patient coded, and a medication was needed—*stat!* The unit clerk called pharmacy for the drug and said: "I need drug _____ STAT! for patient so-and-so in bed . . ." Pharmacy responded that they were busy and had no one to deliver the drug.

The unit clerk frantically replied that there was no one free to run to pharmacy, and an argument ensued. The consultant herself rushed to pharmacy and told them that a patient had coded and needed the drug. A pharmacy tech ran the drug to the unit. The consultant stayed and met with the pharmacy staff and the director who said that if the clerk had explained that a "coded patient" needed the drug, he himself would have delivered it.

This is an excellent example of the difference patient-centered communication would have made had it been the norm of the institution. Instead, efficiency fell victim to egocentric communication and a lack of teamwork. The result was poor patient outcome, substandard management and leadership, and self-centered care. These were problems the consultant had been called in to resolve.

Self-centered or departmental-centered communication—the I's have it—is typical and is often the root cause of intra- and interdepartmental rivalry. A simple shift to "the patient," or better yet, "our patient" terminology would help eliminate that rivalry and improve cooperation. But making the shift is not so simple because we human beings tend to think of ourselves first. For example, we often start by saying, "I need. . . ." We often leave out the specifics of what we need and why we need it. In the above stated case, the unit clerk neglected to say the patient had coded.

Discussion and Application to Practice

In this vignette, misunderstanding between two essential departments—nursing and pharmacy—could have endangered a patient. Simply replacing the word *I* with the words *the patient* would likely have changed the paradigm. Think about the following questions and suggestions:

- Start counting the numbers of times you use the word "I" in a sentence—spoken and written.
- Practice substituting the word *patient* or *we* for *I*.
- Have you ever tried to think of yourself as "the other guy?" Imagine trading places with the patient, a support staff member, or an interdisciplinary team member.
- What steps might you take to shift to patient-centered thinking? Be specific.
- How about patient-centered communication? What might you do to define it and adopt it?
- Again, be candid: do you consider nursing and nurses to be more important than other services? Include in your consideration pharmacists, physical and occupational therapists, social workers, radiation techs, physician assistants, lab techs, and other professionals and paraprofessionals.
- Do you think nursing gets the respect it deserves?
- Do you get the respect you deserve?

NURSE/PHYSICIAN COLLABORATION, COMMUNICATION, COOPERATION

A master's prepared Caucasian advanced practice nurse (APN)—with expertise in coronary care—came upon two Asian PGY-1 resident physicians executing CPR on a hospital visitor who had suffered cardiac arrest. Noting that the MD applying chest compressions had his hands placed several centimeters below the sternum, she knelt beside them and quietly repositioned his hands. The code was a success, and the patient was transferred into the Coronary Care Unit (CCU) with the APN and the two MDs in attendance.

After everything settled down, the physicians severely chastised the nurse for "daring" to correct them publically. She was extremely upset and went to see her CNE to describe what happened. The CNE called the chief of medical affairs (COM) and arranged an immediate conference. The COM listened carefully and paged the doctors, asking them to come to the CNE's office where they defended their behavior. They boldly stated that the nurse was not responsible for patient outcome—they were. They said she had made them "lose face" by correcting them publically.

Cultural differences both simplified and complicated this situation. The relatively easy part was a show and tell—showing them the state's Nurse Practice Act. From this, it was clear that the APN was accountable for patient outcome as long as she had the knowledge to diagnose and treat actual and potential health care problems. In this case, the resultant health care problem would likely have been death.

The cultural element was trickier. Obviously, they knew they were in the United States, a country that at least theoretically puts women on an equal footing with men. Nevertheless, there are many men from certain cultures and countries living here who may not understand or accept this. As a result, the CNE and COM stuck to discussing behavior. Simply stated, the PGY-1's behavior was unacceptable and would not be tolerated. The two physicians may have lost face, but the confrontation ended without hard feelings. One reason is that the APN had not demanded a public apology. She accepted their apology in the relative privacy of the CNE's office before the meeting ended in order to re-establish patient-centered collegiality.

Among other lessons, this vignette points out how important it is to be able to refer to the nurse practice act of your state. In Chapter 10, we will analyze the legal definitions of nursing as well as what nurses say when asked what they do. Nursing is a fine art based on science. It is an important profession, one that is needed everywhere and by everyone at one time or another. Yet, many patients, and sadly many nurses, cannot define what it is nurses actually do. This advanced practice nurse, by her actions, defined nursing well—and was chastised for it. Her director and the chief of medicine backed her. By their actions, two PGY-1 resident physicians were afforded an unusual learning opportunity.

Do you think ignorance of the nurse's role is widespread among physicians, as well as among other health care professionals? What about among nurses, administrators, patients, legislators, and consumers? If you do believe ignorance is widespread, what have *you* done about it? What do you think *should* be done about it?

The encounter reported in the previous vignette was an unusual one. Yet nurses and doctors regularly work together in tight knit clusters. Is there mutual respect? Is there tolerance? Is there distain? Deference? Admiration? How about all of the foregoing? Or, as my economics professor used to say—It *depends*. With some physicians, it does not matter how skilled a nurse is. To them, no one meets the lofty level of a physician except another physician. No one, that is, until a really good nurse pulls that doctor's feet from the fire.

Discussion and Questions to Ponder As You Think About Application to Practice

- Are there circumstances under which you would or would not correct physicians, even if you knew they were wrong? If not, why not?
- What might you have said or done if MDs chastised you the way they reprimanded the APN?
- Do you know the legal definition of nursing for your state? If not, learn it. The ANA Social Policy Statement Appears in Chapter 10 of this book. Use it as a reference. Check out the Scope of Nursing Practice at your place of employment. Know your rights and responsibilities under the law. Practice nursing as a profession, not as a trade. Be proud of what you do.
- Do you believe you would have been supported by your administration, as the APN was in this example?

NURSING/FAMILY MEMBER COLLABORATION, COMMUNICATION, COOPERATION

A 65-year-old man who had recently undergone a quintuple bypass awakened at home with chest pain. His wife, legally blind, called 911 and then contacted her sister—an RN—and asked her to meet them at a local hospital. They met at the ER and expected that they would be permitted to stay with the patient—now extremely agitated—throughout the assessment process. They were wrong. The rules got in the way. Patients over the age of 65 were to be assessed without family intervention, even if the patient requested it. The RN asked for professional courtesy, explaining that the patient could not give an adequate history on his own. He depended on his wife to do so, and she, due to her blindness, depended on her RN sister to join them at the hospital and help them maneuver through the red tape.

The more she talked, the more officious the supervisor became. She finally called over a large security guard who was a moonlighting county police officer. He quoted the rules and forced the RN out of the unit. But she managed to call out to her brother-in-law, instructing him to ask the doctor to allow his wife and sister-in-law to return.

That is what he did. The same supervisor who had them ejected had them readmitted a short time later. The RN asked her if she was embarrassed. She denied that and insisted she was just "following the rules."

Think about rules that:

■ Constrain you in your place of employment.
■ Constrain your patients.
■ Constrain their visitors.

Do you ever make exceptions to these rules? If not, why not?

I saw a bit on TV the other day. A sign over an ICU stated: "No visitors under the age of fifteen."

A mother appeared with her 11-year-old son. She asked to gain admittance. An argument ensued. The ICU nurse said the rules were clear. The mother said the boy wanted to say goodbye to his dying father. "Nevertheless, he is under 15," said the nurse. "But," said the mother, "the boy wants to see his father for the last time. He will not make a scene."

What would you have done?

Many ICUs have rules that allow visiting in 15-minute intervals every several hours. What if your loved one was terminally ill and actively dying? Would you not want the rules stretched so you could be there at his final breath? Some nurses allow for that. Some do not. For them, rules prevail.

Some parents climb into the crib of a dying child. Some nurses want them to climb out. Rules or broken hearts—which are more important? Reading this book, you know my answer. But would you still feel that way if you were on a busy unit? Remember, empathy is an attitude that takes no additional time.

NURSING/VENDOR COLLABORATION, COMMUNICATION, COOPERATION

Not all hospital stories reflect negative experiences. For a change of pace, here is a positive one.

Shortly after taking over a nursing service, a CNE met with all levels of staff. It was the first time in the history of the institution—a hospital/nursing home combination—that professional licensed personnel and unlicensed assistive and entry level personnel were invited to the same meeting.

The CNE introduced herself as an existential manager, one whose philosophy was to be both staff- and patient-centered. Then she asked if there was anything anyone wanted that would make their work life easier. After a moment or two of hushed disbelief a NA raised her hand. Once called upon, she explained that when visiting a friend who was a patient in a nearby hospital, she noticed an aide using a shampoo tray while washing a patient's hair. She said such a tray would be very useful for chronic respiratory patients and others too ill to be showered.

The CNE promised a response to this request within a week.

The next day, she personally called a vendor with whom she had a long-standing professional relationship. He checked with his supplier and delivered a dozen such trays the following day. The CNE asked the nurse managers to hand deliver the trays to those units that needed them. Finally, she personally contacted the NA who had requested them to thank her for her input.

Each tray cost $16.95.

This episode generated the first meeting of the newly formed Product Evaluation Committee. Philosophically, the CNE believed in power to the people. One way of imparting power was giving them decision-making ability over things they used in their everyday work. So she collaborated with the director of materiels management to establish a committee to evaluate products for various factors. These included effectiveness, price control, aesthetics, and usefulness, among other things. Everything from washcloths and underpads to syringes and higher tech equipment went on the product evaluation list. Formation of the committee was congruent with the products to be evaluated. Refreshments were served, and participation was valued. Over time, expenditures went down, and a sense of control and importance went up. It became a win–win situation for all concerned. The new CNE had hit a bases loaded home run.

I have found that the quickest way to break the ice with a new group is to provide something good to eat and get them something they need or even perceive they need. The CNE in the above vignette, by quickly responding to this easy-to-accommodate request—shampoo trays—offered concrete proof that she took seriously both her staff's concerns and her patients' well-being. By asking the nurse managers to bring the trays to the units, she included them as a part of the staff-centered management team. Now the hard work was to begin. Think about what would have happened if she did not follow up as she said she would. Also consider the disappointment and resulting anger if this was a "one shot deal."

Discussion and Points to Ponder as You Think About Application to Practice

Let us take on the entire organization as a point of discussion. Having a new CNE is an enormous change. It can be very threatening. It shakes the foundation of what is and has been the bedrock of daily life for an entire workgroup and, by extension, a workforce and a population of current and future patients. Now there is a new boss, and rumors have been flying. Human nature being what it is, the negatives have outweighed the positives. People are edgy. Although the workers feel safe because they are "protected" by union membership, change is always threatening. Nonunion employees are protected only by their history and perceived value to the organization. Everyone likes the status quo. They know what to expect, so there is perceived safety. But now, there is someone new at the helm, and the deck is bound to be shuffled.

The new leader is also facing some pretty intense challenges. She has been hired to correct many deficiencies, and she does not have a lot of time in which to do so. First, she has to win over her staff. Being a practical-minded person, she knows the staff has been rudderless and that previous leadership, as well as some of the remaining supervisors, have been authoritative and punitive. There has been little input encouraged from staff, especially lower echelon staff, and systems have been practically nonexistent.

The first thing she wants to do is send the message that she considers them equal as human beings. That was the reason for the inclusive meeting. She then wants to give them a voice and provide trust. So she asks them what they need and then gets it for them—shampoo trays.

She also asks them to be empathetic and existential—to walk a mile in the shoes of their housekeeping colleagues in the long-term wing, the nursing home. There, the NAs had not been following protocol to eliminate bulk feces from linen before sending it down chutes to the dirty linen room. She asks them to spend an hour there.

This becomes part of the annual mandatory in-service and orientation, and it solves the problem. The existential manager then turns her attention to the professional staff. Unit by unit, manager by manager, and leader by leader, she evaluates their effectiveness.

There is plenty of room for improvement. A timeline is established for them to boost their performance. Participation in formal management workshops is mandatory. Those in leadership positions without advanced degrees are expected to enroll in college and attend regularly until master's degrees are obtained. This is all accomplished empathetically. Remember—empathy is an attitude that takes no additional time.

Those who cannot or will not participate are invited to apply for reassignment to nonleadership positions. The pathway to success is made clear. Individual needs can be discussed, and programs and outcomes can be modified accordingly. Harshness is not the goal. The objectives are personal, as is professional development and advancement in patient-centered care. Mentoring is offered freely and willingly.

Here are some questions to consider when working to achieve these goals:

- How would you break the ice with a newly assigned staff person?
- Would you take a different approach to elevate the standards, as discussed above?
- What would be your first step if the other staff members were hostile to the newcomer? (Assume upper management allows you choices.)
- What would you do if upper management occupied your time with redundant meetings? Would you just attend or specify your objections?
- What are some actions you might take? Be specific.

At a subsequent NAs meeting coffee and cake were served to entry level staff for the first time ever. The kind of cake was left up to the food services department. They sent a tray of sliced pound cake. When the meeting was called to order by the newly appointed patient-centered/staff-centered CNE, a NA raised her hand. "This cake is not as good as the cake you served to the management staff at their meeting," she said.

Momentarily taken aback, the CNE examined the cake. The NA was correct. Having several choices, the CNE could have said:

A. "I didn't specify the kind of cake when I ordered it. This is what dietary selected."
B. "Cake is cake, and this is the first time you ever had cake served at a meeting." (The implication here is that the NA should not complain.)
C. "Thanks for pointing this out. Next time I'll make equality a point of reference."
D. "Why are you taking up the time of the group with minutiae?"
E. Other.

Consider the same scenario, except that staff members are not comfortable in their management environment, and they do not trust their new boss. They therefore do not feel free to speak up and register their dissatisfaction with the cake. So instead, they pass around notes in a stealthy manner which diverts their attention from the meeting.

The CNE becomes increasingly tense and annoyed, and this sets the tone for future encounters and relationships. From the NA staff members' perspective, they believe that their new boss undervalues them, especially in comparison to the professional management staff. After all, they got better cake. Also, because they were concentrating on communicating with each other, they heard little of what was discussed. The meeting's message becomes distorted, and when it is discussed later in the hallways, it bears little resemblance to what actually was said.

Amazing what a little cake can do.

Whether your staff is welcoming or hostile, keep your focus and language patient-centered. This is particularly important with an antagonistic or threatening individual or group. You cannot go wrong if you do not allow yourself to be diverted. Remember, you are there to improve patient care. To do that, you need a well-functioning team that keeps their eye on their subject of importance—the patient.

Meeting Redundancy

We bring together the best ideas—turning the meetings of our best managers into intellectual orgies. —*Jack Welch*

We all know what an orgy is—it usually has sexual connotations. But for the purposes of discussion concerning meetings, here is a more pertinent definition: an orgy is a period of excessive indulgence in a particular activity or emotion—especially something that has an element of self-pity.

I have had many conversations with nurse managers—those from the middle and those from the top, and I repeatedly detect dread (self-pity) attached to the word *meetings.* Many of these individuals have described some of these meetings as a waste of time, redundant, boring, tedious, and repetitive. It makes me wonder how many of these people have had a sit-down with their bosses and articulated the degree of interference these meetings have with their ability to do their jobs and to further patient-centered care.

I have asked. They have answered—darn few.

Here are a few questions for you:

- Have you assessed and analyzed a cost/benefit ratio for these meetings?
- What do you get out of these analyses?

■ Is there a less time-consuming way to obtain the information imparted at these meetings?

■ How much input do you have? How many nurse managers must attend?

■ Remember the most important question—have you discussed your opinion with your boss? But before you do, read on.

Apply critical thinking techniques to this problem. That is a topic, by the way, that we will cover later on in this book. But do not just sit back and *not* deal with the issues of meeting redundancy. Both patients and staff need your expertise. They depend on you to mentor, counsel, evaluate, demonstrate, lead them, and sometimes run interference for them. The question is: how can you accomplish all this if you are always at meetings?

UNION/MANAGEMENT COLLABORATION, COMMUNICATION, COOPERATION

Strikes are the epitome of conflict within a work environment. Unions have been known to block food, linen, personnel, essential equipment, and materiel from reaching sick babies and other patients normally dependent on caregivers now walking a picket line. Sometimes these individuals call their employers names. Sometimes they target their nonunion colleagues as well. If you have brought in temporary employees—strike breakers—woe be unto them as they walk across the lines.

Think how hard it must be for managers to traverse these boundaries without becoming angry with the staff members who have established them. Imagine what it must feel like to welcome picketers back once the strike is over.

It can also be difficult for staff members on a picket line who do not want to be there—those who believe that management has treated them fairly. They are compelled to participate even though they consider themselves valued and cared about by a management team who listened to their thoughts, complaints, wishes, and suggestions.

There is an axiom in labor relations that goes something like this: a *patient-centered/staff-centered* management team will make for an easier strike. Management has time before an impending strike to remind union-represented staff and nonrepresented staff that they are members of the same team with the same goals—to care for *their* patients. When the strike ends, they will come together as members of one *patient-centered* team. Therefore, it is in everyone's interest to not bring shame upon themselves or their organization.

You might even tell them stories about some Japanese workers who take such pride in their organizations that their strikes are token walkouts. They want to make their point, but they do not want to harm their organization.

However, these techniques only work if they are true. Words are empty unless history and prior action back them up. The time to start a staff-centered management program is not right before an impending labor action. The stage must be set long before that. It might even prevent such actions—but not always.

Sometimes, despite staff-centered management, forces occur that are beyond your control. For example, your organization might be part of a large conglomerate that is facing a strike, and you are caught up in the conflict.

Whatever the situation, remember that the people on the picket line are your staff members. One day, the strike will end, and they will come off the lines to rejoin your patient-centered team. So visit *your* staff members on those picket lines and see to their well-being. Bring hot coffee in cold weather and cool drinks in the heat of summer. This approach can go a long way toward keeping the peace.

But strikes are only one part—a rare occurrence—of union/management interaction. Union-represented workers and management usually are on the same side—that of caring for vulnerable patients. We are on the same team. We work for the same employer. Nurse managers are responsible and accountable to those patients, and they cannot do it alone. It is in everyone's best interest to develop a well-functioning team of diverse individuals and bring them together as cogs in a wheel.

In order to accomplish this, first they must get to know their team members—as individuals. Who are they? What motivates them? What are their work habits, their skills? Consider their strengths, personality types, proclivities, and weaknesses. People have different needs, but one thing is universal, and that is the need for respect.

Bad management means disrespectful management, and this opens the door to hostile relationships with union delegates who believe they must protect their members. This is not as simple as it sounds because one person's idea of respect may be taken as disrespect by another. Suddenly, you are confronted by a hostile union delegate. When that happens, here is a mantra for you: "No appointment—no meeting!"

Do not relent. Hopefully, you have been schooled by your human resources (HR) department or others in interpretation and implementation of the contract. You will know what to do. What you should *not* do is drop everything and meet with the delegate without preparation—no matter how insistent or threatening that delegate may be.

Use the *phonograph technique*: keep repeating the same words—"I will not see you without an appointment. Please return to your work area." Do not give in.

Events like these happen rarely. In the chapter on labor relations, we will discuss contract interpretation and other important related issues. In the meantime, remember that union members are a part of *your* staff. Treat them as such, and include them in your staff- and patient-centered approach.

Discussion and Points to Ponder

- If you work in an organization in which staff is represented for collective bargaining by one, two, or even three unions, it is essential for you to have copies of the contracts and to understand those issues that pertain to day-to-day operations.
- Getting involved in contract negotiations, preparing the contract and related activities is extremely helpful. This aids in developing fluency in interpreting and applying those contracts.
- Involvement is also helpful in developing skill and comfort in preparing for grievance and discipline activities, but it is not enough. Discussion and role playing are important adjuncts that should be conducted with a labor relations/HR expert before you are called upon to actually participate in such activities. Remember, patient-centered care and safety is at stake. You do not want unsafe practitioners at your bedsides.
- Make sure you understand the concept of the management rights clause, as well as the contract language that states: "All other duties and responsibilities as assigned. . ."

This common clause in union contracts gives management personnel the right to assign workers to duties and responsibilities not specifically spelled out in the contract. This does not mean management can ask a NA to lay bricks. It does mean management can ask a worker to do something new within a job classification—such as add cleaning toilets to a housekeeper's job responsibilities. In so doing, management must take into consideration staffing and the extra time it takes to clean toilets or make empty beds after discharge cleaning. In general, job descriptions belong to management. Prudent management discusses changes with the union, since a good working relationship should be cultivated. They do not, however, ask permission. The phrase, "the union won't let us do it," has no place in a well-run, patient-centered organization.

Now, ask yourself:

- Have you established and maintained staff-centered relationships?
- How do you know?
- Do you know and care how it *feels* to be your subordinate?
- What is it like to be a patient on your unit?

In my consulting experience, the vast majority of managers I have worked with on labor/management issues have never seen a contract, much less been instructed on its clauses or interpretation in the workplace. This makes them helpless in the face of intimidating employees or delegates telling them some things are either "not my job" or "not in the contract," or words to that effect. If that happens to you, pull out a contract (or job description) and ask the employee to point out the effective clause.

WALK A MILE IN MY SHOES

Some organizations have a *walk a mile in my shoes* day, during which some staff members actually shift roles. This can be a real eye-opener if your subordinate is willing to imitate your behavior. Until that happens, some of us really do not know how we come across to others. As a substitute, try a round of unit conferences—wear masks, serve cake (I'm back to that again) and have a little fun. Humor in the workplace has been proven to ease tension and increase productivity. It even lowers blood pressure. If people are honest with you—or even if they are not—the question of how it *feels* to be your subordinate may be answered for you.

Here is how one CNE used humor to make her point.

She was the nurse executive of a world famous diagnostic center. Sometimes members of the Board of Directors—very powerful individuals—were extremely demanding. She often carried what she described as a "magic wand" to board meetings—you know, the kind you can get at Disneyland. When members of the board and medical executive committee asked too much of her, she would toss it on the table and say: "Here, this has stopped working for me, maybe it will work better for you." This quickly broke the tension building in the room.

To get back to the question of how it feels to be your subordinate, or a patient on your unit: these questions are trickier. If I were a unit manager, I would talk to my staff members and to my patients and ask them. Then I would listen. As a consultant, I have done just that and have found that people love to talk about their experiences as long as they do not fear retribution. Some have been pleased, while others have been visibly frightened. Interestingly, but not surprisingly, there were several universal themes to staff members' concerns. At all levels, they complained about disrespect, dishonesty, unfairness, untimeliness, and the like.

Patients, too, had certain themes. These included waiting for pain control meds, the food, incessant noise, and rude, uncaring staff. I have heard these issues articulated by my friends, people on buses, people on subways and by people in Starbucks who have talked. The stories I have heard are what motivated me to write this book. I wish I had heard stories of good, caring experiences, but alas, that is rarely the case.

FLIRTING IN THE WORKPLACE

Is flirting a form of collaboration, cooperation, and communication? Is it harmless fun, or insidious? When does it cross the line and become harassment? Is it an individualized perception? You decide.

There was a support service personnel strike. I was the patient care administrator at the time. Volunteers from a local nursing college provided relief care. Suddenly, there was a commotion caused by a rush of all male administrators to the ramp leading from the parking lot to the ER. I went to see what was attracting them.

A sweet young thing wearing a mini skirt had sashayed across the picket line and was gliding sensuously toward the ramp. She was braless under her form-fitting T-shirt, and her long blonde hair swung provocatively with each step. Watching the men watching the young woman was an interesting stress-breaking activity during a difficult strike. But, as with all things, it had a beginning and an end.

As she entered the building, I ushered her into an ER cubicle where I obtained a set of scrubs and a loose-fitting lab coat for her to wear as her uniform of the day. I then counseled her about professional comportment and attire.

The administrators returned to their work assignments. In this case, it was clear that no one felt harassed, but let us kick it up a bit and make the student nurse a female nurse manager who was on a unit and got too close to a subordinate nurse. As she leaned over him or her—provocatively—she demanded he work an overtime shift which he did not want to work.

There is a fine line between flirting and harassment, and it is often in the minds of the people involved. Most would agree that the student nurse was flirting. What would make it harassment? Perhaps if she were in a power position and her behavior caused discomfort to a subordinate. The higher the power/discomfort ratio, the greater the likelihood that it qualifies as harassment. That said, the greater the power of the harasser, the more likely it is that the victim will become upset and blow the whistle. That could trigger a lawsuit—or worse.

Here is another example: an employee health physician was known to add breast exams to his preemployment physicals. Is this flirting or sexual abuse? Or is it a necessary part of the preemployment physical? One day, a potential employee objected. He threatened her with denial of employment if she persisted in her refusal. She brought him up on charges of sexual harassment. During the investigation, other employees came forward. They had all felt abused but feared repercussions if they complained.

The physician—a contract employee—had his contract terminated and suffered other penalties. Unfortunately, the employees subjected to this harassment started their jobs with a negative experience, as opposed to feeling welcomed. One can only hope that staff members and patients were not subjected to similar behavior on the patient care units. The truth of the matter, however, is that human beings are sexual creatures, and flirting is part of human behavior. It is important that management develops trusting relationships with staff, so that they feel—there is that word again, *feel*—comfortable approaching their manager if they believe they have been threatened by sexually charged behavior.

The ABCs of Patient-Centered Care: A—Administrative; B—Board; C—Collaboration, Cooperation, and Communication

I am going to conclude this chapter with the letters A, B, C, but before I do, let us play a letter game that involves the letter P for philosophy. David Brooks of the *New York Times* wrote an op-ed entitled, *The End of Philosophy* (2009), in which he compares Socrates—who believed moral thinking requires reason and deliberation—with modern, cognitive scientists who see moral thinking as a matter of aesthetics. We *see* and we *evaluate* simultaneously. Reason and deliberation are not necessary to draw conclusions.

Brooks quotes Steven Quartz of the California Institute of Technology, who said during a recent ethics discussion sponsored by the John Templeton Foundation, "Our brain is computing value at every fraction of a second . . . What our brain is for is to find what is of value in our environment."

Carry this into our world of nursing and health care, and into patient-centered and concomitantly staff-centered care. We know what it is and what it is not. We know it when we see it. We do not have to process it—not even for a second.

We also know that to implement any philosophy, Administration, the Board of Directors, and the Chief Executive Officer must generate and support it. They must all "walk the walk" and "talk the talk." One would think that those at the top would model the brand. But in all the places I have visited, and all the well-meaning nurses, doctors, academics, and administrators with whom I have spoken, I have heard lip service instead of authenticity given to patient/staff-centered care. Too often, professional nurses are diverted to accomplish tasks better left to unlicensed support personnel.

I cannot explain why the industry persists in wasting money in so egregious a manner. It truly is penny-wise and pound-foolish—in the long run—to have RNs running errands, answering phones, wasting time at duplicative meetings, doing clerical work, and accomplishing a myriad of mundane tasks more efficiently left to others. Freeing them would allow RNs to focus their time on professional nursing care—on diagnosing and treating actual and potential health problems, restoring function, and saving lives. Instead, many professional nurses waste time and money working below their capacity and pay category. The ongoing need for communication, collaboration, and cooperation with those at the top is greater than ever as we move deeper into the twenty-first century. Health care reform at the bedside is no less important than it was in the Halls of Congress.

SUMMARY

This chapter concerns itself with the importance of creating positive empathetic, collaborative/cooperative relationships between and among the various entities within the health delivery environment. These include nursing staff and patients, nursing staff and leadership/management, nursing team members, the interdisciplinary team, nurse/physician, nursing/family members, nursing/vendors, and union/management.

▪ Understand the importance of cooperative, positive relationships among and between management/leadership and patients and staff. Attitudes are contagious. They flow downhill.

- Praise publically, criticize privately; except in emergency situations. Try to role-model, mentor, and correct—not criticize.
- Realize the importance of *asking* staff and patients how it *feels* to be a part of the organization and your unit—as well as how important it is for leadership to set the tone and direction for patient- and staff-centered philosophy, goal setting, and implementation.
- Shift from egocentric communication—the *I's* have it—to patient-centric communication—the *patient* needs it—or the *unit* needs it to enhance communication, cooperation, and collaboration.
- Bring supplies and equipment to point of service whenever and wherever possible. Do not waste precious staff time searching for supplies and equipment.
- Improve listening skills to enhance communication and establish trust.
- Develop relationships with A—Administration, B—Board, and C—CEO.

CHAPTER ENDNOTES

American Nurses Association. 2009. Nursing Administration: Scope & Standards of Practice. *ANCC Magnet Recognition Program.* Silver Springs, MD: American Nurses Association.

Brooks, D. "The End of Philosophy." *The New York Times*, April 6, 2009. http://www.nytimes.com/.

2

The Organization: Shifting Authority and Communication From Top Down to Patient Centered

Every company has two organizational structures: The formal one is written on the charts; the other one is the everyday relationships of the men and women in the organization. —*Harold S. Geneen*

Opening Vignette

The scene: board room of an acute care medical center.
Participants: directors of all patient care and support service departments and the administrators to whom they report.
Presiding: CEO and CFO.
Subject: staff cutbacks.

Absent From the Agenda: Patients

Fiscal discipline and reimbursement reduction issues at health care facilities have recently been major topics of concern. In view of large deficits, health delivery organizations have been decreasing their expenses in order to maintain viability and avoid closing units or their doors. This gathering is the first step in what is expected to be a long process of meeting these fiscal crises head on.

The CEO opens the conference and quickly hands over control to the CFO. She uses slides and PowerPoint demonstrations to drive home the rather dismal outlook. Drastic measures must be taken to alter the landscape. The air is heavy with concern as department heads shuffle their thoughts to meet the crisis. They are wondering, "Is my job safe? How many layoffs will there be?" The one question missing is: What will be the impact on patients?

Eventually, the CFO turns the floor back to the CEO. Without missing a beat, he stands up and switches the lights back on. He returns to his seat, looks around the table and says, "OK, it's your turn. We need a 10%

personnel cut from every department by the end of the week. Take most of it from education and administration, assuming you have those positions to cull from. Then work from the top down.

As everyone at the table starts to object, the CEO and CFO get up and head to the door. Immediately before leaving, the CEO turns and emphatically says: "There will be no appeals—just do it!"

Everyone rushes back to their offices. The CNE stops at the CEO's office on her way—they are both in the administrative suite. He is in a meeting, and the door is closed. She leaves a handwritten note urging him to allow her to meet the fiscal burden using her own judgment as to whom to let go. Her rationale is patient-centered. She wants to make cuts that will have the least impact on quality of care.

She hands the note to the CEO's secretary and says she will return from a prescheduled meeting in 1 hour. When she does, she finds a termination notice on her desk. With it is a note from the CEO stating, "I told you there would be no appeals."

This CNE was employed by the organization for 4 years. All her performance appraisals were more than satisfactory. There was nothing in her record that indicated any dissatisfaction with either her work performance or interpersonal relations. But this was a new CEO, and shortly after the CNE was terminated, he brought in a CNE with whom he had worked at his former place of employment.

There is a Latin saying that means: "The thing speaks for itself." It is appropriate to use here: res ipsa loquitor.

Here is another vignette that describes a similar scenario in that it occurred during the same fiscal crisis, and it was at a meeting of departmental directors headed up by a CEO and a fiscal consultant. These two individuals demanded that a group of leaders and administrators cut services to save money. The administrators of the patient care and support service divisions, both relatively new to the organization, prevailed upon the CEO to allow them time to *enhance* patient care delivery and amenities in an effort to boost admissions, thereby increasing revenue. The CEO was skeptical but agreed to a trial period.

The CNE had already improved patient care services through augmented education and mentoring of all nursing personnel levels. She also established high professional management standards and deliberate replacement of substandard staff with ambitious, upwardly mobile, professional nurses. Existing managers were involved in leadership training and rose to elevated standards of practice. It was time to market these changes to the medical staff so as to encourage them to step up their admission rate to the facility.

Support services had improved care of the physical plant and raised the quality of the soap, body lotion, linen, and cleaning supplies. Both the hospital and nursing home had raised the standards and products, clinically and physically.

In order to spread this news, the CNE, as a part of her regular patient rounds, asked patients how they felt about the care they received. When she got positive responses, she asked them, if they wished, to write her a note when they got home. When she received such a note, she routinely:

- Mailed a thank you note to the patient.
- Sent a letter to the admitting physician along with a copy of the patient's note.
- Posted a copy of the patient's thank you note on a prominent bulletin board.

Admissions soon increased, as did staff satisfaction. Layoffs and other cost-saving measures were averted.

A footnote: Two other hospitals, at which the fiscal advisor consulted, followed his advice to cut staff and services without consulting heads of departments. Both hospitals eventually closed their doors.

Res ipsa loquitor.

As we segue into the organizational shape of many health care organizations today, keep the real focus of health care in mind. Specifically, to whom are we referring when we say health care? If it refers to our patients—then why does the word patient not appear in the organizational chart?

What follows is a letter written by a patient, now deceased. Her daughter—a former director of nursing and a friend of mine—found it when going through her mother's papers. This patient gives an account of care that was cold and inhumane. She asks the same question I did in the previous paragraph, perhaps in different words and in a different place, "To whom do we refer when we use the term health care?" Since the organizational chart gives no clue, we turn to this former patient—Anna Kleinfeld—for the answer. She states it most eloquently:

The Grand Edifice With No Heart

I leave for Florida for the winter and my cousins start their daily routine of driving me to their house almost every afternoon. We play cards, gossip, and then have a delicious gourmet supper and [they drive me] back to my motel.

The night of December 29th I do my usual chores of washing my panties and stockings, but I find myself getting up about four times that night with a dull ache in my chest. I take a nitro each time and go back to sleep until it is light.

Shall I call my home doctor in New York? The answer will surely be to go to a local doctor! Shall I wait it out myself? Don't be a wise guy! I phone my cousin—he has a heart condition—hoping his doctor will see me. Instead he says: "Get dressed, he will see you at Emergency." I find the waiting room full of people. It's 8 a.m. I don't think I even had my orange juice, and lately, crowds sort of confuse me. No doctor, just questions after questions after questions, perhaps except why I was born.

My mouth gets dry just when a set of young men appear with yellow pads to be filled out with answers to questions—the same questions already asked.

There is one little Indian girl in pigtails who smiles, so I whisper: "Does anybody read all this?"

She whispers back: "It's for the records."

So can't one set of questions and answers be put through a computer in this wonderful age of technology and be distributed to those interns?

I am foggy, confused, and don't even know if I'm in pain anymore.

A doctor finally introduces himself. By this time I don't remember anything he asks. I am completely drained. It must be after lunch because I ask for a cup of tea and get it, and I get into a bed.

Then the fun begins. Cardiogrammed, X-rayed, and blood drawn—and blood drawn again. At one point they take blood from the same arm within an interval of a few hours. I don't realize it or that my arm goes dead and will stay dead for many days. No one speaks, never a smile. Just hustle and bustle and everyone starched and proper.

It is New Year's weekend and two nurses are assigned for the two women in my room. As one is fixing the other woman I say, "Nurse, please give me something I cannot reach," because I was gated on both sides. And the answer—"I am not your nurse—I am only assigned to this one."

The new medicine does not agree with me and the pain starts. My new doctor and the resident definitely agree it is not a heart attack. By now I realize I just had too much steak the night before.

The medicine must have been changed because the pain starts again—in my arms and spreads to the nape of my neck and just roams all over my torso down to my wrists. All my blood running through my veins is on fire. I ask one of the nurses for help one night. She says she will call the doctor. All night I sit up and rock my body. I have my own Nitro that I take occasionally; I lie down for a while but soon have to sit up again.

By the time the doctor arrives the next day I am so exhausted, bewildered, I don't know what I say, or what he decides to change, but the pain lessens. Always I wait for the beginning of those horrible pains in my arms.

Again I am to go to X-ray. The orderly whizzes me away. I'm a little alert. The floors are shining marble, and my goodness, the plaques on the walls. Donations, donations. I am sure many were given by the parents of those beautiful interns. Soon I am going so fast I hold on tight not to fly away, and I hear muttering in back of me. "Damn, this is good when I have time to flirt with the nurses—not running those chairs all the time." But most of all the aloofness, the starchy proper mien on everyone that sort of goes with the shiny floors and brass plaques.

I think I stay eight days and then go home with my daughter where I really have a heart attack. But let me finish—I am crying out before I completely forget it all.

Remember, you are a house of healing. We are not live cadavers. With your next donation buy a very large machine and spray your marble floors with the milk of human kindness and let everyone, everyone from the highest to the lowest step into it. If by a miracle this gets into the right hands and your attitude changes, I know my road to oblivion will be paved with stars.

Amen,

Anna Kleinfeld (88 years of age)

I wish I could say this was an unusual experience, but I am afraid that would be untrue. Anna Kleinfeld is only one of a multitude of patients who suffer at the hands of uncaring staff. Remember, this book is meant to help us look at our failures and correct what is wrong.

That does not mean we should not celebrate the many things we do exceptionally well. As an example, I have included the account of Jacquelyn Burns, MS, RN, Nurse Leader M15, Memorial Sloan Kettering Cancer Center. Jacquelyn's story is featured in the Epilogue. She epitomizes the qualities of leadership, empathy, expertise, good humor, flexibility, sympathy, charisma, and a reverence for human life. Jacquelyn is representative of many nurses who provide exceptional care to thousands of patients every day—nurses like the CNE in the opening vignette in this chapter, who lost her job as a result of her patient advocacy. Fortunately, she went on to a better job in a more prestigious place. If she had to do it over again—to advocate for patients—she would. How do I know? She told me so. But good does not excuse bad.

DOES FORM FOLLOW FUNCTION, OR DOES FUNCTION FOLLOW FORM?

This is an old, familiar question—one that is particularly important to the health care industry when designing an organization. If you examine the structure of most health care organizations, you will routinely see a hierarchic shape. In this model, individuals with the most power—the CEO,

administrators, and department heads—are at the top, in the power positions. The lower down you go, the less power you have. In the diagram
below, the boxes represent administration and the various departments.
Straight lines connect the boxes. These represent direct lines of command
and communication. You will also see broken lines connecting department
heads and others. These represent lines of communication and cooperation.
The problem with this hierarchical shape is that authority and communication flows top to bottom, and no matter how many broken lines appear on
the chart, internecine rivalry is a human condition. You do not have to look
very hard to notice that the patient is absent from this diagram, and often
from conversation.

Two other organizational shapes that may appear both in the literature
and in practice are pyramidal and matrix. Pyramidal is just what it sounds

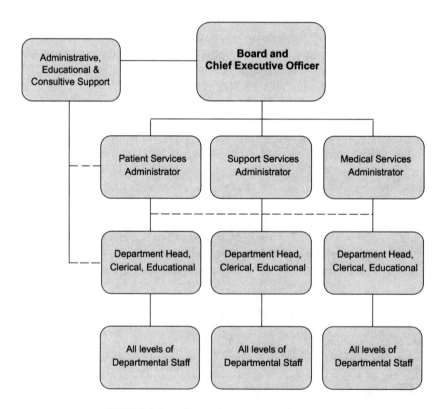

FIGURE 2.1 Hierarchical organization chart.

like—shaped like a pyramid. But it has the same problems as the one previous, since power flows from the top, interfering with direct-line communication. Also, that all important patient is missing from the chart. Matrix shape—not to be confused with trademarked Matrix Management©—makes the effort to bridge the communication gap between the top and the bottom by stretching out the organization and creating something like a flattened beehive or an uncoiled geodesic dome. This one also features top–down lines of communication, although not as steep, and it still fails to focus on the patient.

Because I found the existing shapes unsatisfying, I created another model—one that has not been represented in literature, but one I have used for teaching purposes. As you can quickly see in Figure 2.2, it has the patient as its central focus. Nursing—the 24/7 department—surrounds the patient. All other services access the patient in cooperation and collaboration with nursing.

This often happens anyway, but having a visual model in many ways sanctions and institutionalizes the relationships. The use of organizational charts goes back a long way—in fact, it goes back a very long way.

According to *The Executive Fast Track (2008)*, the Egyptians were the first to employ an organizational diagram to illustrate the division of labor

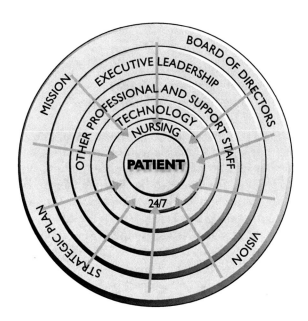

FIGURE 2.2 Concentric organizational chart.

on their greatest project—the construction of the pyramids. Now fast forward to 1855 when Daniel C. McCallum (1815–1878) introduced them to
this country by way of the railroad industry. He used them for the same
purposes as did the Egyptians—and as do we—when supervising the Erie
Railroad construction in New York. His charts included lines running from
superintendants to subordinates within divisions—while keeping those divisions separately structured. They were neither too dissimilar from today's
tree-like structures, nor were his communication methods. The superin-
tendents wrote weekly reports to their supervisors who reviewed them and
gave instructions that filtered downward.

The Erie railroad and McCallum's charts and communication methods became a model in this country. Remember what I said earlier in this chapter:

■ Power and communication flow from top down
■ So said the Pharaoh in ancient Egypt and
■ So say many of our CEOs in today's health care establishments.

CHANGE IS SLOW—BUT KEEPING THE SAME FORMAT FOR CENTURIES: HERE IS SOMETHING NEW TO CONSIDER

In the concentric chart depicted in Figure 2.2, patient-centered care is improved because of:

■ Availability of team members to patients.
■ Proximity of team members to each other.
■ Decreases in the patient's sense of vulnerability.

But the improvement takes place only if the visual model is applied by
assertive, skilled nursing professionals who transpose the visual representation into a concrete actuality of care. The circular pattern can then become
a cocoon-like safety net, implemented by staff members whose attention is
internally centered on patients and laterally focused on teammates.

But it is not just nursing that is responsible for safe and sound patient-
centered care. It is the job of everyone in the organization, especially those
at the top leadership level who set the tone. They model the organization's
vision and mission—or they should. The question is, do they?

Ask yourself if and when—in the past week, month, or quarter—you
have interacted with your immediate supervisor. Then, ask yourself the
same question, but replace immediate supervisor first with your CNE, then

with your departmental administrator. Now kick it up to the CEO and even to the board member with responsibility for your department. Now add the patient to the mix—after all, that is why you are in business. Have you seen any of these people on the patient care units? How often? What were they doing? That is right—what were they doing?

Remember the example in the opening scenario. There, the patient was admitted to an oncology unit in a world-class hospital but could not get immediate care for a bleeding wound. There, an RN said she could do nothing without medical orders. The patient saw the CNE on the unit once during a week-long stay, but her attention was focused on a video camera instead of on patients or staff. Why? Because a TV station was interviewing her about her preceptorship program for new grads. She spoke glowingly of all the support these new grads received and of a patient-focused philosophy.

At the same time, the patient was being discharged by an RN with longevity at that hospital. She commented that it was the first time in months that the CNE had been seen on that unit.

. . . IN YOUR EXPERIENCE . . .

Have you had these kinds of experiences? Have you interacted with your CNE on your unit of assignment? What about the other individuals in your hierarchy? Is your only contact with them at meetings or through memos? Your answers to these questions will reveal the kind of organization for which you work. But you likely already know.

Vignette Up the Achievement Ladder

Here is another revealing vignette. It demonstrates the philosophy of a staff nurse, promoted to nurse manager, promoted to CEO.

The CEO of a two-hospital division within a large health system conglomerate was in an elevator with three men who she referred to as "the suits." They were top executives from the corporate office visiting her two facilities. The men were heading from the first to the fourth floor. The elevator stopped unexpectedly on the third floor and the door opened to reveal an elderly patient crying as though her heart would break. The CEO moved to block the elevator door from closing and asked the patient what was wrong. Sobbing, the patient begged for a Coca Cola. The CEO asked "the suits" to meet her on the fourth floor while she dashed to the third floor nursing station and cleared the patient medically for the requested drink. She then rushed to the coffee shop where she obtained the soda, hurried back to the third floor, and handed it to the patient. She then ran to floor four to rejoin her startled companions. About 5 minutes had elapsed from start to finish, and patient-centered care had been accomplished.

Discussion and Points to Ponder as You Consider Application to Practice

Can you imagine your CEO, CNE, or immediate supervisor dropping everything in order to satisfy a patient's request? Would you go to such lengths?

Now, consider this scenario: A CNE of a skilled nursing facility received word that the son of one of her nursing assistants (NA) was shot dead in the mean streets of a major city in which crime rates were high. The NA was being informed of the incident by a friend in the staff locker room. The CNE dropped everything and ran to the locker room just as the NA collapsed to the floor. The CNE got down on her knees and cradled the NA's head in her lap and wrapped her arms around her, cooing to her as though she were a child. The NA was in a state of hysterical collapse. Emergency rescue was called.

The CNE remained with the NA as she was transferred by ambulance to a local ER, where she stayed with her until family arrived. Then, she returned to her facility. Word of her caring concern spread like wildfire throughout the organization, but she had not done it for notoriety. She was a caring person, concerned for the well-being of her patients, as well as the staff members who attended to these patients' needs.

Here are some points to consider:

- Would have behaved this way given the opportunity and the power?
- Have you ever felt someone else's physical, emotional, or psychic pain so deeply that you were moved to tears?
- What did you do and how did you do it?
- What did you want to do that you feared doing, if anything?

In the Eye of the Beholder

The following situation took place at a seminar about a concept known as *Culture Change*. This refers to altering a long-term care facility's entire atmosphere, ambiance, and care model from a traditional medical model to a system known as patient-focused care. Here, all personnel are educated and oriented to place the resident at the center of attention for all they do. They, the patients, are in charge of their time and destiny. They rule their roost as though it were their home.

The change takes place over time, and the physical plant is altered to accommodate the new model of care and concern. Ideally, residents live in clusters as would a small family; meals are served when requested, baths or showers are provided as asked for, recreational activities are individually tailored, and the like. Plants, pets, music, outings, and other activities of active living replace the dreaded environment of nursing homes of the past—where residents await death and often receive it as a release from an unwelcomed life.

But this is not what the tour groups saw on their rounds. Despite upbeat guides pointing out new window curtains and buffet tables in institutional-like dining rooms, staff members gathered at nursing stations and residents sat apathetically in chairs or lay diagonally across their beds with a shoe or two hanging from their feet. Indeed, in this place, culture change was in the eye of the staff and not in the realm of reality. This brings us again to the shape of the organization and the conduct, nature, general behavior, interaction, appearance, and disposition of individuals within it. In other words, how did they behave and interrelate within their organization?

Organizational behavior according to Lamb-Deans at Cornell University ILR School:

> *This is the study of individuals and their behavior within the context of the organization in a workplace setting. It is an interdisciplinary field that includes sociology, psychology, communication, and management. Keywords include Organizational Behavior, Organizational Change, Organizational Development, Corporate Culture, Corporate Communication, Group Behavior, and Human Decision Making.*

Let us take these one at a time and apply them to the health care organization.

Organizational Behavior

How people communicate and act within an organization depends on the kind of organization in which they work. Is it military or religious? Is it authoritarian or *Lassez Faire*? What are its missions and goals? What are the communication styles of its leaders and managers?

Organizational Change

Remember this: Master plans impede success. It may sound cute, but in general, the only person who likes change is a wet baby or the person holding the wet baby. The message here is that implementing change is a process to be undertaken slowly, over time, and with the input and cooperation of those concerned and affected by the change. People and organizations will likely resist change—even change that improves their lives.

For a good example of organizational change, look into the Eden Alternative in the long-term care industry (Eden Alternative, 2009). This model has irrevocably altered—for the better—the long-term model as we know it.

Having consulted with organizations undergoing organizational change to an Eden-like model, with a goal to reach this or similar models of care, I have seen the before, the during, and the after effects. Like a rubber band being stretched to a new shape, organizations—comprised of human beings—resist change—all kinds of change. Given time, encouragement, and repetition, however, the new shape starts to become the norm. Patience and consideration, involvement and empowerment all help to dispel resistance.

Organizational Development

The focus here is on improving individuals within the organization as a means to improving the entire organization. In-service education, mentoring at the bedside, literature reviews, and journal clubs, are all ways to develop individuals within an organization. Without ongoing development, people and organizations stagnate and then contract.

Corporate Culture

Culture refers to shared values, assumptions, and norms. Corporate culture refers to these same things shared within an organization or a corporation, and it does not take long to identify the culture. Walk into an organization and see if you feel comfortable or uneasy. You will probably sense it before you know it. Notice how people are dressed. Formally or casually? Is there a sense of importance in the way people move and do things? How about small groups—are folks hanging out, or do they seem to be engaged in active communication? What does the physical plant look like? All these and more comprise the corporate culture. Think about what you might add to the list.

Corporate Communication

This refers to internal as well as external communication. Are there newsletters, memos, and meeting minutes? Is communication respectful? Is proper English spoken, or are slang and colloquialism the accepted means of speech? What mechanism is there for feedback up the hierarchy? What about down and across the organization? How about to and from the community?

Group Behavior

This refers to behaviors people might engage in as part of a group that they might not participate in as individuals. These might be positive or negative. Elsewhere in this book, I relate a story of a union official riling up a group of social workers into an angry mob. This is an example of negative group behavior. A similar example would be violence on a picket line. The opposite might be when someone with charisma and influence enters an area in which violent action is taking place and calms a situation down. Think of a town hall meeting where tempers are flaring and someone with persuasive capability—or a big gun—comes along. The thing to remember is that the group does not always reflect the individuals within it.

Human Decision Making

You could spend an entire course of study on this fascinating topic. If you have ever served on a jury or had to decide whether or not to buy an expensive car, you know how complex a process it is to come to a decision.

The question to be answered here is—what resources are available within the organization to assist you in making the *right* decisions in serving patients wisely and therapeutically? Are there reference materials handy? Can you reach an educator if you need one? What about your supervisor?

Will you obtain mentoring without fear of criticism? Have you refined your critical thinking skills?

ORGANIZATIONAL STUDIES

The basis for organizational studies is to explain, predict, and control human behavior in the context of the work environment—the organization—in an effort to enhance productivity. A seminal study of human behavior in an organizational construct is the noted Hawthorne study, which describes what is known as the Hawthorne effect. This study was conducted at Hawthorne Electric Company where, in order to boost productivity, lighting was changed. Indeed, production improved. Over time, production flagged, so lighting was returned to its former level. Because human beings crave and respond to attention, production once again improved.

We know this from observing child behavior. Children will do almost anything to get attention—even negative attention is better than no attention at all. Workers will do likewise and so will patients. After all, they are human, too.

Recently, I watched a program on The Learning Channel, a segment of which showed a 4-month-old infant interacting with its mother. At first, the mother cooed and smiled at the baby, who responded happily and actively. Then, the mother averted her eyes, folded her hands in her lap, and paid no attention to the baby—or to anything else. At first, the baby tried to engage the mother by gurgling, slapping the table, and smiling. But soon, the baby became still, sad, and depressed. It reacted negatively to attention being withdrawn.

People respond positively to positive attention and negatively to negative attention. But they also react negatively to no attention. Remember this as you develop your leadership style—a subject we will discuss in detail in the chapter concerning this issue.

EFFECTIVE COMMUNICATION—AN IMPOSSIBLE GOAL?

Vignette   Blintzes for Brunch

My husband and I went to our local diner for brunch. Since it was a holiday weekend in celebration of Memorial Day, I decided to splurge and order one of my favorite dishes—cheese blintzes with sour cream and cinnamon. I like them crisp on the outside with a creamy filling. The chefs at the diner tend to place the blintzes on a bed of lettuce. The lettuce causes moisture to form under the blintzes, making them limp. So I asked the waiter to have them served without lettuce. He acknowledged my request.

Soon, our order arrived. If my blintzes had been served as I had ordered them, you would not be reading this. In fact, they were nestled deeply within a bed of freshly washed lettuce. Sighing, I quickly removed them and placed them on a napkin, patting each one gently to absorb the moisture. As I did so, I muttered, "Doesn't anyone listen anymore?"

In truth, listening is an art, and active listening—what I call listening, hearing, and absorbing what is said, and then responding appropriately—is both an art and a science. Unfortunately, we often find it missing from both our social and professional lives.

Our patients tell us many things—it is too hot, it is too cold. It hurts, it feels good. It is lonely, it is uncomfortable. I am afraid. Our staff members also tell us things, both overtly and subtly. But do we really hear what they are saying? Do we listen with our third ear?

As you go through this chapter, think about these things. Put yourself in positions of control and loss of control. Remember that to communicate effectively, we must listen effectively. This may sound elementary, but it is oh so complicated, and it is the gateway to all other forms of effective communication.

To listen means to pay attention. But what does communication—in its entirety—actually mean? The etymology of the word "communication" or "communicatio" (in its Latin form) contains two root words: com (for the Latin "cum," which translates to "with" or "together with") and unio (Latin for "union," from which our English word communicate directly comes). Therefore, communication refers to union with or union together with. Two other words—community and communion—come from the same base words. All mean to share.

Take a look at the word communion in the religious sense. It actually means to take in the body of the deity—to become one with God. In the most effective, existential form of human communication—in the phenomenological sense—we can only strive to become one with our patients in the patient-centered care environment or with staff members in the managerial relationship. In the first case, communion with our patients enables us to seek a deeper understanding of the patient experience *from the patient's point of view.* In the second case, it is to ask ourselves or our staff members what it *feels* like to be a member of our team.

My 104-year-old stepmother Mim (now deceased) was a resident in an assisted living facility. One day, she was asked by a health department surveyor, "How do you feel?"

Mim responded, "I feel with my fingers. How do *you* feel?"

Don't you think this is a pretty nifty response for a 104-year-old? But we in the caregiving community do not have the luxury to feel *only* with our fingers. We need to feel with our hearts and minds as well.

PRATFALLS AND PITFALLS OF COMMUNICATION

Give an oral instruction and expect a negative result—if not immediately, then soon. Add an accent, and it will be sooner. Add a speech or hearing deficit, or ambient noise, or distraction, or a hurried or impaired mind, or a myriad of other things, and the negative results will far outpace the positive. Someone will eventually suffer a harmful outcome as a result of the negative communication. Quite a conundrum—isn't it? But it sounds like a sure fire thing to me. So let us begin with the process of communication and segue into patterns of miscommunication. Then, we will see what can be done to improve outcomes.

Evaluating the process of communication is easy. The organs of articulation must be intact. The farther off center—or normal—they go, the greater is the likelihood of error. These include such things as the mouth, tongue, teeth, glottis, epiglottis . . . you get the point. Then there is hearing and the brain. You are nurses, so think of anatomy and physiology and fill in the rest.

Next is the space in which or on which the communication is to take place—what is the medium? Is the atmosphere noisy or nice? How is one's handwriting, and the reader's eyesight? What about using a computer? You know the questions to ask. Oh, and do not forget commonality of language. You cannot speak Greek to an Englishman and expect understanding. Even when people are multilingual, there is context and idiom to consider. Then there is body language and social space. The words, "I love you," accompanied by an angry grimace and a raised fist do not convey the same meaning as when accompanied by a smile and a pleasant demeanor. And remember to stay away from definites. Try to not say words like *all* and *every*, and remember, there are exceptions to most rules.

To help you in this game of trying to perfect communication skills, here are a few examples concerning miscommunication patterns. Let us begin with "Inference/Observation Confusion."

Inference/Observation Confusion

Professor and author William V. Haney, a well-known researcher, professor, and consultant, developed a test known as the Uncritical Inference Test (Haney, 1973). It involves making a conjecture while believing something had actually been observed. Haney relates the famous case of General George Patton, who, during World War Two in the European Theater of Operation, slapped a soldier for malingering. The General, a rough, tough, fighter, *observed* the soldier in sick bay and actually *inferred* that he was lazy. After he left the area, the soldier was found to have high fever, and there was proof that he had malaria.

Not too many malaria cases going around? Here is a more mundane example. You see a young woman wearing a necklace just like the one stolen from your mother last week. Without another thought, in the company of a large group of people, you accuse her of stealing your mother's necklace. You are totally embarrassed when she shows you—and them—proof of purchase.

What Had Happened
You *observed* the necklace around a stranger's neck and you *inferred* she had stolen it. Worse yet, you *acted* on your *inference/observation*.

Here is something that actually happened to me. I entered a diner and saw my father at the counter sharing his meal with a buxom blonde. Momentarily struck speechless, I pondered my options. I could rush out and notify my mother. I could ignore the whole thing. I could confront my father and the blonde. What would you have done?

This is what I actually did. I walked over to the couple and said, "Hello," to my father. He turned and greeted me without any concern and introduced me to the blonde as someone he had just met. He said she had asked if he liked his fish, so he had offered her a taste. This rang absolutely true to me, and I sat down next to my father and ordered coffee. No harm, no foul. But think of all the damage I could have done had I converted my observation into a different inference—and then acted upon it.

Here is a nursing example of Inference/Observation Confusion: A white male patient fled a psychiatric facility and ran through a white neighborhood. Two African American male orderlies gave chase. The neighbors called the police, who arrested the orderlies and allowed the patient to escape. Is this a good time to say *res ipsa loquitor*?

According to Haney, *bypassing* is another element of these same "patterns of miscommunication." Here is a nursing example: A nurse tells an aide to give a patient a bath—meaning a bed bath. The NA puts the patient in the tub. Who is at fault?

As Haney notes, words can have multiple meanings. As an example, he takes the word fast and uses it as follows: to run *fast*; or to travel in *fast* company; a watch is *fast* when it is ahead of time; a person can be *fast* asleep; to refrain from eating is to *fast*; color is *fast* when it does not run; a person can play it *fast* and loose; a racetrack is *fast*; to eat breakfast is to break one's *fast*; etc.

Here is one of my favorites—read it aloud for best effect. It is an anonymous poem that Haney calls "the piling on of usages," and you'll also find it on the Internet in varying formats:

> *Remember when hippie meant big in the hips,*
> *And a trip involved travel in cars, planes, and ships?*
> *When pot was a vessel for cooking things in,*
> *And hooked was what grandmother's rugs may have been?*
> *When fix was a verb that meant mend or repair?*
> *And be-in meant merely existing somewhere?*
> *When neat meant well-organized, tidy, and clean?*
> *And grass was a ground cover, normally green?*
> *When groovy meant furrowed with channels and hollows,*
> *And birds were winged creatures, like robins and swallows?*
> *When fuzz was a substance real fluffy like lint?*
> *And bread came from bakeries and not from the mint?*
> *And roll was a bun, and rock was a stone,*
> *And hang-up was something you did with the phone?*
> *It's groovy, man groovy,*
> *But English it's not.*
> *Methinks that our language is going to pot.*

And I think this is a good segue into the next section.

WORKPLACE HUMOR OR THE LAUGH'S ON WHOM?

According to Randy Erickson, President and CEO, National Association for the Humor Impaired, known as Dr. Humor, workplace humor is good for workers, customers, and for overall business. All the same, working people tend to think and act industriously and seriously, both about what they do and how they do it. But is this necessarily a bad thing?

What Are the Facts?

Recent research has shown that incorporating humor—especially laughter-producing humor into the workplace—is a good thing. Laughter eases tension and exercises the lungs. This, in turn, increases oxygen in the bloodstream, and we all know that oxygen feeds the brain. Now, we have a workforce that is alert and happy. Even better, laughter lowers blood pressure and improves a sense of well-being by increasing endorphins.

There are some caveats when planning to incorporate humor into your work environment. Obviously, sensitivity must be maintained, and remarks about race, religion, and physical characteristics are off limits, and there are other more delicate, potentially hurtful subjects. Remember that the goal is to cultivate a staff-centered and, ultimately, a patient-centered philosophy and environment. To do so takes finesse and infinite patience—over time.

In bringing humor into your work environment, be careful to not be rude, crude, or sexist. I recently learned of a gynecologist's office in which its all-female staff had papered its waiting room with cartoons depicting men as comic creatures of ridicule. Some were downright obscene. The word unprofessional was the kindest term that came to my mind.

I remember, as a very young nurse, being oriented to a labor and delivery unit. As the head nurse was showing me the med station, a physician walked past the desk and said hello. I knew something was off, but I could not put my finger on it. Cookie, the head nurse, started to giggle. "He does that to every new nurse," she said. Does what? I asked, puzzled. "Puts his leg on backwards." She responded as she laughed out loud. The doctor had left his leg in Korea and had adjusted well to the loss. He could make a joke of it. But it would have been rude and crude coming from anyone else.

Humor need not be lewd or dirty. It need not pick on someone's appearance, body parts, or something else personal about them. Try starting each meeting with a clip from *I Love Lucy* or dress in something funny or even silly—try a clown nose at a management meeting. How you dress up can be subtle: Top off your hair with a wig close to your hair color but slightly different. Say nothing until someone else does. Or it can be outlandish—a purple Mohawk perhaps. Change your usual attire—pantsuits to long skirts, or scrubs to business suits. If you work on pediatrics, it is easier to come to work dressed like Mary Poppins than if you work on med/surg—but you do get the point—right?

Peds and geriatric units are great places on which to inject humor. Just be sensitive to how patients react and be ready to break off if you are not getting what you expected. If your empathy meter is turned to high, you will not have a problem with staff members, patients, or even your boss. Stick with the mantra—empathy is a feeling, an attitude. It takes no additional time.

Another way to inject humor is to rent movies from a well known consultant like John Cleese of *Fawlty Towers* and *Monty Python* fame. I had the pleasure of seeing him—on tape—when *Nursing Spectrum* integrated a program of humor into its human resources development program. We laughed until our stomach muscles hurt and tears ran down our cheeks. But no one complained of a headache or a nervous tic for a very long time after that series was aired.

THE HARDER THE JOB, THE GREATER THE NEED

In the final analysis, the harder the job, the greater the need for respite. As previously discussed, many nurses have told me they do not have time for the bathroom, much less to take a rest break. As existential managers, we do have time to bring some humor into our work environments. All we need is to give our imaginations room to breathe. Give it a try, even if it means turning your lab coat inside out and wearing garish flowers in your lapel. You can always duck into a restroom on your way to one of those infernal meetings to sort yourself out. If nothing else, at least your staff had a good laugh before they had to go back to business.

Questions and Points to Ponder for Application to Practice

Bearing in mind that most health care organizations are hierarchical with communication flowing from top down, how can you—the middle manager—ensure both receipt of and proper dissemination of undistorted, timely information? As a corollary to the foregoing question, how can you ensure that your staff understands and can apply concepts from that communication?

Here is where you have power—you are the boss of your unit. Use all the means of communication you have available to you—message boards, unit conferences, minutes with a signature line for those who were absent. Use the Joint Commission rule: If it is not written, it is assumed to have not been done. Most importantly, get some feedback. Talk to your staff. Just hanging minutes on a bulletin board and asking staff to initial them does not mean the information they contained was absorbed. In fact, come in from the negative point of view—assume it was not absorbed. That is right—make that assumption until you validate otherwise. Remember, though, what that word *assume* does when you break it down to its essential parts: The old adage is that it makes an (ass) out of (U) and out of (me). Always validate!

BITS AND PIECES

So many bits and pieces of information come down from on high that really are meaningless to the operational, day-to-day life of the business. So, take the plunge. You decide what you *should* emphasize and what you should sit on.

You report feeling stressed. This new program—humor in the workplace—is an added burden. Your nurse leader does not think she has time to help you—but she has been told it must be implemented, so she has passed it on for you to do. You have been given no choice in the matter. What are your options?

At first, do nothing. Sleep off your feelings of despair. They will pass. The bottom line is, the boss says, "Do it," so, eventually you will have to do it. Once you are a little more rested, seek out someone in the organization with whom you have a good, empathetic relationship. Ask this person to help you work out an approach. Make it fun. You will soon get in step. As a practical person you have to—so you might as well enjoy it. Here is one approach.

Even though you are sick and tired of being expected to do more with less, you have already thought of something yourself. You have asked to be allowed to incorporate the housekeeping staff into your unit staff, only to be put off. Nevertheless, you have already won their cooperation and loyalty. The housekeepers sit in on your unit conferences and participate. The dietary staff—when they deliver food—manage to take a seat and join in because you have established a welcoming environment. It is good for your patients. It is good for you.

Once you obtain approval from the support services hierarchy, you hope to have all support staff work together making unoccupied beds, interacting with patients, handing out tissues or a drink of water. But then one day you are reprimanded for these activities. What happened?

After you recover from the shock you feel—you write a response—carefully, didactically, and academically. Use before-and-after statistics. Make it a time and motion study. Show how you have freed up professional nursing time by using less expensive support staff time. Housekeeping and dietary have taken up some slack. The unit is cleaner, and satisfaction levels have improved among staff and patients. Use of linen and central supply products have decreased, so costs have been trimmed.

This program has become a win–win patient- and staff-centered success. Now it is up to you to sell it to the boss.

SUMMARY

In this chapter, we discussed individuals as they relate to each other in the organization. The focus throughout was to shift authority and attention from top down to patient-centered.

- Typical health care organizational charts are hierarchical (Figure 2.1) (or pyramidal or matrix) with communication and power flowing from top down—rarely is the patent depicted on the chart.
- A concentric organizational chart (Figure 2.2) is presented as an alternative. This depicts the patient at the center, like the hub of a wheel, with nursing as the 24/7 service surrounding the patient. All services and departments are shown as the spokes of a wheel, interacting with nursing to access and care for the patient—collegially with nursing.
- Effective communication requires a complex series of useful competencies: listening, speaking, and writing clearly; nonverbal communication, not confusing observation with inference, ensuring feedback to prevent bypassing, and validating comprehension.
- Ensure a free-flow of communication—not just downward in direction.
- The physical, psychological, and emotional value of humor in the workplace equates to increased productivity, decreased turnover, and improved patient and staff satisfaction.
- Overcoming resistance to change takes time and effort—without which there can be no progress.
- Recognize what is important then prioritize.
- Use the Joint Commission rule: If it is not written, it is assumed to have not been done.
- Most importantly, obtain feedback.

CHAPTER ENDNOTES

Eden Alternative®. http://www.edenalt.org. (Cited 2009).

Haney, W. V. 1973. *Communication and organizational behavior text and cases*, 3rd ed. Homewood, IL: Richard D. Irwin, Inc.

McCallum, D. C. http://en.wikipedia.org/wiki/Daniel_McCallum (accessed April 14, 2010). Daniel McCallum (1815–1878) was a railroad engineer and manager. He became the General Superintendent of the New York and Erie Railroad in 1855, and then founded the McCallum Bridge Company in 1858. He was an early proponent of the organizational chart as a way to manage business operations.

3

Leadership/Management—Can You Tell Them Apart?

Management is efficiency in climbing the ladder of success; leadership determines whether the ladder is leaning against the right wall.

—*Steven R. Covey*

Vignette A CNE—A Stranger to Many; Known to Few

"Some of you may not know me because you work nights and weekends," she said as introduction to the first around-the-clock staff meeting held in nearly 6 months. Apparently oblivious to the snickers in the room, she picked up a preplanned agenda and concentrated her attention on it, discussing the impending Joint Commission survey.

Staff members became restless. They fidgeted in their seats and checked their watches. Some dozed; others yawned or scribbled on note pads. Had she looked up from her notes, she might have realized that she was wasting her time—and theirs. Her voice had a droning quality, better suited to relaxation tapes than to a nursing staff meeting.

Finally, the hour-long session was over. She looked at her watch and mumbled, "No time for questions."

"Thank God," someone muttered as the staff fled the room. It was unlikely that anyone retained much information. Fortunately, this was a seasoned group of people that had been through many Joint Commission surveys before and would likely ace this one. Their time would have been better spent in a give-and-take dialogue with their director. But she seemed hell bent on not engaging in discourse. Perhaps she feared getting to know her own staff, or maybe she dreaded hearing about problems that she then would have to solve. Whatever it was, we know that it was not an example of good leadership. In the next story, we see an illustration of creativity. There are lessons to be learned from both.

Vignette   The "TION" List

The facility was old and tired. Its patient population was elderly, and many individuals suffered with varying degrees of senile dementia. They were being prepared for an eventual move to a new facility, but their memories were unpredictable. Those with good recall were nervous and upset about being moved from the only home they had known for years.

All RNs not wanting to transfer to the suburbs had left for other jobs. Nursing administration was therefore working with per diems and angry nurse aides (NAs) who did not want to make the move either. But they were trapped by seniority issues and an inability to find other jobs.

On the positive side, the NAs cared about their patients. They had been with them for a long time—in many cases, for decades. Nevertheless, just about everyone was miserable—except for the new nursing director and a newly hired assistant director—me. She had taken a chance and hired me despite my lack of posted qualifications. I had always been sure of myself and my ability to learn quickly. But I was a little anxious because my new boss told me that the health department (HD) was coming in 2 weeks and I was to "clean up" the charts.

Health Department visits to long-term care establishments were a new experience for me—but I had heard about them and the power that they wielded. I turned to the NAs for help.

Meetings were scheduled and refreshments were served—a new experience for them. Nevertheless, I was greeted by a scowling and suspicious group of disgruntled people sitting around the table with arms folded tightly across their chests. They belonged to a "tough" union and had never had anything but insincere and combative encounters with management.

After introducing myself and asking them to do likewise, I pushed to the center of the table a large tray of cake and invited them to partake.

At first there was silence. Then an aide reached for a piece as I poured coffee and passed the cream and sugar. Finally, they relaxed in their chairs, and I discussed the HD visit and asked for their cooperation.

A few looked skeptical. So I explained that I understood their concern about new bosses and the move to a new facility. I encouraged a response. A few spoke up, then more. The ice was broken. I shared my goals, which were to:

- Get to know the staff as quickly as possible, and have them get to know and trust me.
- Quickly become familiar with the patients.
- Get the charts ready for inspection.
- Above all, ensure patient-centered care.

I looked around the room and saw suspicion, doubt, hope, skepticism, anticipation, and everything in between. I decided to ignore all the looks and move ahead. Sometimes, a little *in*attention goes a long way.

We ended the meeting and headed for the patient units, dropping an aide off at her unit along the way. I stayed with the aide on the last unit and visited each patient, reviewing my prepared check list for essential health issues. I called it my SHUN or *TION* LIST:

- AmbulaTION
- SocializaTION
- MentaTION
- OxygenaTION
- NutriTION
- EliminaTION; and so on

I made unit rounds with the NA who knew the patients best and assessed each patient against each TION. I used patient-centered terminology and complimented each aide when appropriate. This way, I was able to write a valid nursing assessment and open lines of communication that had been previously closed. Now I had to keep them open.

MANAGEMENT DEFINED AND OPERATIONALIZED

Management is generally defined as *leading, organizing, directing,* and *controlling a workforce toward an organizational goal.* In nursing *management*, the ultimate goal is patient care excellence. Here is a list of *leadership* qualities needed to reach management's goals. If this sounds like both a conundrum and a challenge, it is. Remember, a leader can lead to any goal; a manager leads to the organization's goal.

Leaders mobilize, motivate, liberate, facilitate, release potential, and pique the interest, energy and commitment of the workforce, so it—or they—can achieve the organization's goals, if they choose. They might choose otherwise. For example, as we shall see in the chapter on collective bargaining, they may prefer to pursue the union's goals, and remember, as we saw from the opening vignette: *Leadership is action, not position.* This highlights the fact that there are both formal leaders—the ones with the titles but not necessarily anything more—and informal leaders, the ones with followers.

Organizing is management's next task. Check out your pantry at home. Can you find the ketchup? "Oh," you say, "That's not fair. My husband, kids, mother-in-law, and even my dog moves stuff around. Ask about my unit at work—not something at home." (Look for more about dogs in Chapter 4—Labor/Management).

"OK, what about the supply closet or med room, or . . ."

But you might say that is not fair either because so many people have access to that as well. That is true but. . .

"What shall I ask about?"

As the manager, you are responsible to see that your staff has the supplies they need—on hand—when and where they need them.

Not fair? You say. You are not in control of supplies and equipment? Well, what exactly *is* under your control?

Let us start with the language.

Have you noticed that the small words in English sometimes carry the heaviest weight? Words like ***but, only, so***, *of*, and *if*. Watch for these words. In the case of supplies—wrest control, give your staff—all your staff—input and have your supply and linen closets set up as suggested. Then, educate your staff and others to follow established patterns ***so*** patient-centered and staff-centered care can be accommodated and maintained. In the long run, everyone will be accommodated, ***but only if*** everyone has been socialized to focus on the goal ***of*** patient-centered care. Sounds simple? It's not. At first, someone has to police the area and the process. Someone has to mark the shelves. Someone has to obtain cooperation from other departments. Someone has to validate pars and keep them updated, and I sincerely hope that someone is not you—the nurse leader. Your job is to agree or disagree that whoever is doing it is doing it correctly, so your staff can readily obtain for your patients what they need when they need it—24/7.

Now use language, statistics, and your new patient-centered care philosophy to solve your patient-centered care problem. Isolate and identify. Start with the worst first. What are the negative outcomes? What would solve the problem?

Use your computer and double check your work. Make sure your English and math are accurate and inform your director in advance. No one appreciates surprises, unless it is a party.

What you do not want to do is remain helpless in the face of problems that reduce patient-centered care to below the standard *you* have established for *your* unit. Take ownership.

Direct and *Control.* These are two heavily weighted words. The question is, would you rather do the directing or be directed? How about control? Control or be controlled? I refer back to my economics professor at Columbia University, who said the answer to every question in economics is, "It depends." So, it is here.

Here are some examples where "it depends" takes on real meaning in life and death issues:

If you were trapped in a raging fire, it is likely that you would rather be rescued by a seasoned firefighter than by a neophyte. But if that expert were not available, you would depend on anyone with the required skills, wouldn't you?

If you suffered a cardiac arrest, it is likely that you would rather depend on a board-certified cardiopulmonary medical specialist to administer CPR than a casual bystander who was certified in CPR. *But* what if that trained MD, or an RN, was not available? Then you would settle for anyone to step forward and try to save your life.

In a patient-centered care approach, the patient *is* or *should be* the focus of attention. It should not *depend* on staffing ratios or other resources. The manager directs and controls resources, and one of the resources is the workforce. It simplifies the issue when you look at it this way.

Recently, when I asked a patient-centered, successful nurse leader about her philosophy and practices, she told me she gives her staff what they say they need and want, including time off and assignment requests. She believes in management by wandering around all work areas, and she mentors at the bedside. She ensures that her staff has, within easy reach, the supplies and equipment required for caring for their patients. I mentioned her before—she is worth mentioning again: Her name is Jacquelyn Burns, MS, RN, and she is a nurse leader at Memorial Sloan Kettering Cancer Center in New York City.

ORGANIZATIONAL GOAL (PATIENT-CENTERED CARE)

We have now come full circle. We have defined and described management as leading, organizing, directing, and controlling a workforce. All that is left to discuss in this chapter is the organizational goal. For the purposes of this book, the organizational goal is *Patient-Centered Care*.

What does that actually mean? In Chapter 2, I introduced a concentric organizational chart with the patient at the nucleus of everyone's consideration. But that is just on paper. How do we make it so? One way is to change our language.

Changing the Language From Egocentric to Patient Centric

It is about an hour into the shift and the phone rings. It is the staffing manager who says to the unit clerk, "I need Nurse So-and-So to go to unit 1-B. Please tell her to get there as soon as possible." She then hangs up and continues her calls, unmindful of the chaos she has unleashed.

The unit clerk finds the nurse and communicates the message. The nurse is in the midst of developing treatment plans and preparing medications for her five or so patients.

She stops what she is doing and groans. She detests the unit to which she has been assigned, and as team leader, she now has to distribute care of her very sick patients to several reluctant and overextended colleagues. One of them is still on orientation and very shaky in her new role. Additionally, a terminally ill patient she had been caring for has finally opened up to her. She has assured him she would be there with him during the shift.

She discusses her concerns with her nurse manager who simply shrugs. She phones her supervisor who snaps, "Just go!"

When you examine the supervisor's behavior and language, it smacks of egocentricity. Her word choices are self-centered and authoritarian—"I" need you to go. She orders her to "just go," rather than using any number of empathetic, problem-solving, participative responses.

A successful, outwardly focused leader understands that dependence on one's followers is essential for success. Explaining why an action was taken leads to understanding. Participation between supervisor and professional, or any member of the workforce, is essential to positive teambuilding and successful outcomes.

In the case of the nurse being reluctant to float—it is not patient-centered to force someone to do anything against her or his will, especially in the type of situation described. Here is an alternative.

Vignette   GWYNs

She was known to be a great nurse leader who championed the cause of nurse middle managers and of RNs in general. As a director of nursing, she knew several things. She knew that patients were best served by empowered RNs who were both challenged and satisfied in their work, and she knew it was counterproductive to compel people to do what they did not want to do. She also knew that when you asked nurses to do more than their peers, it was only fair to pay them more than their peers. So she established a pool of nurses who wanted to float and assigned them a special pay rate. She used the title GWYN for "go where you're needed," and gave each of them embroidered shoulder patches, which they proudly wore.

All the nurses in this pool were cross-trained so they could be called upon to work on any unit. Because there was money and prestige in the assignment, it was not long before there was a waiting list for the pool. No longer did staffing managers have to "pull teeth" to get nurses to float. Those nurses who floated had their eyes on patient-centered care—instead of on a bull's eye on their staffing manager's back. Soon, even the language changed and people were talking about patients' well-being instead of about their frustration. The problem of balancing staffing after start of shift and disrupting patient care was eliminated.

Here is another example highlighting the success of this model: Union-represented support staff in several departments willingly stepped outside their job classifications to lend a hand because of their strong patient-centered care focus. They also embraced staff-centered participatory management styles of an entire middle management group.

Vignette   Ask and You Shall Receive

Five-hundred-fifty debilitated long-term patients requiring skilled nursing care and acute and long-term rehabilitation care were being prepared to move across a large quadrangle from a decrepit building to an attractive new facility. The nursing, building services, dietary, security, and pharmacy directors all had a participatory management style, which led to excellent interpersonal relations with their staff and with each other. They held weekly planning meetings to update each other and prepare for the move.

Support staff was represented by a strong and sometimes bellicose union that constantly reminded union members to not step outside the parameters of their job descriptions. Nevertheless, during staff meetings, when suggestions were solicited from housekeeping personnel as to how to move so many patients in their wheelchairs between breakfast and midmorning snack, they all offered to "handle it." To be clear, transporting patients was not in their job description.

The same was true of all departmental support personnel, as well as the professional staff. Everyone, except for a few outliers, did whatever was needed to both transport the patients and make them comfortable in their new surroundings. The move that top administration anticipated to take the better part of the day was completed in a few hours. In fact, the photographers employed to document the move had nothing to photograph when they arrived. Some patients and staff members had to be asked to pose for photos—which they readily agreed to do.

In short, patient-centered and staff-centered care won the day. This is not to say that there were never any grievances or union–management strife. In the chapter on collective bargaining, you will read about some in this very facility. But on this day, everyone had his or her eye on the goal.

Sometimes, a simple shift from the "I" word to the word "patient" or "we" starts the ball rolling away from egocentric to patient-centric language. Refer back to chapter 1 for discussions about effective communication.

Who Makes the Better Manager?

It is clear, often within the same organization, that some managers do a better job than others. Education, certification, and years of service can be measured and accounted for, but these may not be among the causative factors. Personality, charisma, and respectful consideration, along with leadership style and dedication to patient care, do, however, seem to make a difference. The more outgoing and physically active the manager is, the more she wanders around. The more she wanders around, the more visible and engaged she is with staff members, patients, and others with whom she has contact. This has a direct correlation with improved morale and enhanced patient care outcomes.

Allow me to repeat this vital concept: *The more outgoing and physically active the manager is, the more she wanders around. The more she wanders around, the more visible and engaged she is with staff members, patients, and with everyone else. This has a direct correlation with improved morale and enhanced patient care outcomes.*

But being active and being there is not enough. One must be well grounded in leadership and management theory and, of course, all that goes with these important specialties—and one must apply theory to practice.

That is called *Praxis* and *Praxis Intervention*, which, according to Webster's, is theory applied to practice. The Web service Wikipedia offers a more complete definition (Praxis Practice, 2010). Basically, it is the process by which a theory, lesson, or skill is enacted or practiced.

Praxis is where emphasis is placed on gaining firsthand experience of concepts, intelligent application of knowledge, empathy and sympathy, listening skills, discretion, and a reflective relationship between theories and action. Let us go over these one at a time and see how they relate to great leaders:

- *Gaining firsthand experience of concepts, not only theoretical but perceptive*: *Great leaders* often lead not only with their heads, but with their hearts and souls as well. They seem to have an almost ethereal or other-worldly grasp of what is going on and what makes people tick.
- *Intelligent application of knowledge*: *Great leaders* understand that it is not enough to solve problems and advance the patient care environment, especially in the hectic health care world of today. The perceptive leader–manager must not only have a world of knowledge, but also be able to apply it in a timely, intelligent, and intuitive manner.
- *Empathy*: The *Great leader*–manager cannot turn a cold countenance toward employees, expressing only an imperative to "get the job done!" She must apply knowledge in an intuitive manner and motivate staff to follow her to the ends of time and space.
- *Sympathy*: It is fine to feel sorry *for* one's team members when they are stressed by too much work and too little support, but it is not enough. What good are words when someone is suffering from fatigue and job concerns? The *Great leader* knows that true understanding cannot be feigned. It is either real or the leader/manager will soon be known as the great pretender.
- *Listening skills*: It does not take additional time to listen effectively and give appropriate feedback. You might hear something important that could be costly to you, your staff members, and patients if you miss it. The *Great leader* remembers the lessons of childhood—stop, look, and listen before you step off the curb into oncoming traffic—or into a problem that you have not properly analyzed.

■ *Discretion:* "Loose Lips Sink Ships." The *Great leader* knows that this timeless expression from the World War Two era is no less applicable today. Trust and prudence go hand-in-hand.

■ *Reflective relationship between theory and action:* The *Great leader* thinks about dressing for work or for a date. You look in the mirror and see reflected there something you do not like, so you change it. Then you look again. If you like what you see, you move on. If you do not, you alter it again.

That is a reflective relationship; a deep, weighty, philosophical, insight-ful relationship, not a superficial connection. This takes time and effort, but in the long run, you will find it actually saves time.

Apply these concepts to your relationship with your staff members and you will get to know them at a deep phenomenological level, and with that knowledge comes trust. With trust comes the security of knowing that your patients are cared for properly—that their needs are met; that their chances of being restored to optimum levels of functioning are maxi-mized; that their physical, psychosocial, emotional, and spiritual needs are properly attended to while they are in your care. Do they deserve any less?

Empathy/Sympathy—Differentiated and Defined

Empathy is the vicarious experience of feelings, thoughts, or attitudes of another. It is to feel *with*. When someone is suffering, the empathetic indi-vidual actually feels the pain.

As I write these words, I hearken back to an episode in the original *Star Trek* series about an empath—a creature so empathetic and compassionate that she *felt* the actual pain of an anguished tormented human being. She even developed the physical characteristics of extreme suffering that the human was undergoing.

Sympathy, on the other hand, is harmony of or agreement in feeling—to feel *for*. In this case, the bystander does not actually feel the pain, but feels sorry for the person who is suffering pain.

As we further our investigation into leadership, we will discuss various behavioral styles and consider whether someone must be born with certain characteristics in order to become a great leader. We will look back in his-tory at the impact of charismatic leaders and failed leaders. As you read, ask yourself whether empathy was a part of their humanity—a part of their skill set. Is it part of yours?

LEADERSHIP—DO THE A'S HAVE IT ONCE AGAIN?

As I reviewed this manuscript late in January of 2010, a man entered a jewelry store in a tony neighborhood in New York City. He pointed a gun at two men who stood behind a counter filled with diamonds and other precious gems, after showing the men a fully loaded magazine in his gun. He then demanded that they hand over the jewels. One of the men said "NO!" So the robber shot him dead. He then fled with nearly one million dollars in fine jewelry.

Despite strong authoritarian—sometimes known as autocratic—behavior, it did not work, and someone died. Did that make it evil? The answer is "no." But because its intention was for iniquitous purposes—it fell under the rubric of malevolence. But when the authoritarian leader is motivated by good intentions, its character changes. When a neophyte nurse is confronted with a patient who codes, her supervisor autocratically says "step aside." Authoritarian action is called for in a fire or terrorist emergency, or when a nurse freezes under pressure.

In general, folks do not like to be bossed around—except in a crisis when their lives are in danger. So maybe it is not the orders that make authoritarian leadership bad; perhaps it has to do with goals. When the USAir plane was brought down in the Hudson River, the passengers were glad to be told what to do in an authoritarian manner and style. Following orders probably saved their lives. This was no time for a participatory management approach.

Because I was interested in the action and leadership style that, USAir commander Captain Chesley Sullenberger took, I made it a point to listen to the Transit Safety Board hearings. Captain Sullenberger was asked why he did not instruct the cabin crew to prepare the passengers for a water landing. Remember, he had only seconds to make decisions. He replied that he did not want anyone wasting precious time donning life jackets when he believed that they really needed to prepare their bodies for a crash landing. If they survived the crash with their bodies intact, he said, they could then deal with the next problem. If they wasted precious time struggling with life jackets, there would be no next problem with which to deal.

A great leader is able to make split second decisions and take responsibility for his or her actions. Captain Sullenberger epitomizes great leaders.

He kept a cool head; he was highly skilled; he took immediate action; he made split-second decisions; he thought outside the box; he tread where no one had gone before; he took responsibility for his actions; he had already gained the trust of his team members; and he was the last man out.

Would you have been able to replicate Captain Sullenberger's greatness within your realm of practice? Have you been confronted with situations that have made you uncomfortable? Are you an introvert that has had to assume the role of an extrovert—to be the authority in manner and style?

There are many questions about leadership styles and their appropriate use under specific circumstances. Captain Sullenberger employed an authoritative approach—absolutely essential during emergencies such as the one he encountered.

To help you consider your options under many circumstances that you may encounter, let us take a look back in history and see how others have fared.

Leader Behavior Styles—An Historical Review (Political Leadership Theory)

Leadership discussions have been documented as far back as the early Greek philosophers, upon whom much of our ethical decision making is based. To further our discussion on ethics, see Chapter 9. In the meantime, we can take a look at Plato's and Aristotle's views about leadership.

Plato believed that superior intelligence was essential to effective leadership and that it far outranked physical aptitude and proficiency. He thought that a leader needed to have the capacity to understand moral truths or to create a proper vision of what serves the best interests of the public at large. Without this vision, Plato believed that leaders could not determine how the public should be governed—or led. This thinking—that government was comprised of superior beings and the public as a group was made up of those needing to be led, placed the interests of the state over the interests of individuals.

Aristotle, on the other hand, believed that good leaders must appeal to three things. They must appeal to:

- Ethos—Character
- Logos—Reason
- Pathos—Emotion

An effective leader must demonstrate character and appeal and must build that character among the public or within the group to be led. They should demonstrate reason and should think and act in a logical way. They should also show a human side through appropriate display of emotion.

Also found among Aristotle's beliefs are the importance of:

▓ Intelligence, good sense, and practical wisdom *(phronêsis)*
▓ Good will and respect for the troops (substitute staff) *(eúnoiâ)*
▓ Professional competence and spirited personal integrity *(aretê).*

As one reads ancient philosophy, including Plato and Aristotle, it is interesting to note the foundational wisdom and ease of application to today's leadership environment. Professional competence and respect for the "troops" are vitally important to leadership success. But sometimes, the lack of these essential qualities is incredibly destructive to competent patient-centered care. Sometimes, lower echelon employees are nearly "invisible" to everyone except their peers—and union organizers. Sometimes, RNs are so *needy*, they *need* their morale boosted by external forces instead of feeling a sense of worth in the important job they do. Sometimes, clinical ineptitude slips past a nurse manager and/or a nurse educator and is seen by a patient or a physician, and our entire profession takes a hit. Here is such a story.

Recently, a physician told me he had asked a nurse to double the dose of a nitro patch on his patient suffering ongoing angina. The nurse proceeded to place the second patch directly over the first. I was as disturbed at her lack of competency as was he, but I also was embarrassed that an RN would do something so clinically unskilled—so indicative of a lack of critical thinking skills.

I relate the story here because, somehow, this staff nurse's clinical ineptitude slipped past her manager and her educator. Fortunately, there was no harm done to the patient because the physician caught the error. However, he did not report it to the nursing hierarchy nor did he spend time with the RN, explaining her mistake.

I promised to add his story to my book, and I place it here for you to contemplate as you think about Aristotle's view of competence. Now think about yours.

To move on to other well-known persons who wrote about leadership, the name *Niccolo Machiavelli*, born in Florence, Italy, in 1469, stands out. In fact, the name has become an adjective meaning cunning, crafty, and sly. However, he actually lived his life for politics and patriotism. The reason he is associated with corruption is a small pamphlet called *The Prince*, which he wrote to gain influence with the ruling Medici family in Florence. The political genius of Niccolo Machiavelli was overshadowed by the reputation he was unfairly given because of a misunderstanding of his political views.

When one is called Machiavellian, one is thought of as having acted in a deceitful, underhanded manner.

But remember, nothing really is black or white. Everything comes in shades of gray, and although the ends do not necessarily justify the means, sometimes we do things for the greater good. Machiavelli, it turns out, did not necessarily deserve the reputation he acquired. As is sung in the Gilbert and Sullivan operetta *Pinafore*: . . . "Things are seldom what they seem, skim milk masquerades as cream." In today's food markets, skim milk indeed masquerades as cream: one brand states it is "creamy tasting," "skim plus." That tells us that both the big and the little things—like details—count (as if we did not know)—as I believe it did in the following vignette.

This story is about a final class for a master's in nursing program at a well-reputed university. The professor told her students that they needed to exhibit three things to pass the course.

Vignette   Three Strikes and You Are In

The professor required her students to first demonstrate knowledge of the subject matter. Second, demonstrate application of theory to practice, and finally, prepare a document evidencing these accomplishments with the competency and fluency one would expect of a master's-prepared professional.

All of the students could articulate knowledge of the subject matter and application to practice. About one third could not prepare a fluent document consistent with a high school education, much less a graduate degree. The professor and the students found themselves between a rock and a hard place.

All but one student made the commitment to apply herself to improving her writing skills with the assistance of the professor—an empathetic individual who agreed to mentor the students. An incomplete grade was registered for them and intensive tutoring commenced. Each applied herself diligently and, within the agreed-to time frame, submitted an acceptable paper. The incomplete grade was replaced by a passing score, and they graduated with their classmates.

Discussion: Words and appearance have power—both the spoken word and the written word, which also has staying power. Mastering writing and developing effective presentation skills seems to elude too many nurse leaders and even nurse executives. There is power in knowledge and in a commitment to the professional obligation of lifelong learning; yet sometimes, hostility greets the suggestion that an associate's degree or a bachelor's degree is a starting point, not an endpoint. Some faculty cannot write a professional paper. Can you?

If you are uncomfortable with your writing skills or making a presentation in front of an audience, it is never too late to learn. Keep an open mind and focus on finding programs that make learning fun. But for now, let us spend a moment or two on the sometimes difficult issue of positively handling patient care errors in a patient-centered environment.

Why assume a punitive, demeaning approach? It is not only a dreadful part of our history, but we teach staff members to be cunning and crafty. We encourage them to not only deceive themselves, but also to deceive their nurse leaders and managers.

So how should we approach this? After all, errors are serious matters. Patient safety is at stake. Trust is at issue. We want staff members to come forward and share in damage control. Our goal is for them to seek education and updating without fear of reprisal or embarrassment. We also do not want to tolerate repeat offenders.

There is an old saying that might just illuminate the pathway to enlightenment in this and other sticky management issues:

It's not what you say but the way that you say it
It's not what you do but the way that you do it

Discipline is never easy—even self-discipline. But if you are kind and empathetic and have a magnetism about you, it makes it easier on you, and most especially on your subject. But before we move on to the issue of magnetism—or charisma—think about the words you will choose. Try to keep your discussion to the *act* and not the *person*. It is what the person *did* that requires attention and correction—not the person. The person is not faulty—the act is faulty.

Charismatic Leadership

Now we can turn to Max Weber, who among other things discussed charismatic leadership in 1947. He referred to such luminaries as those persons set apart from ordinary people, specifically referring to Buddha, Churchill,

Gandhi, and Christ. He noted that they and other charismatic individuals had exceptional powers of confidence and were inspirational and attractive to others.

The outstanding question is: Can you obtain charisma, or do you have to be born with it? If you think about the individuals named, they seem to share certain traits—an inner glow, magnetism, a shining light emanating from their eyes. Certainly not things you can buy or otherwise acquire.

Importantly, it should be noted, that charisma does not always come to those in benevolent personas. Think of Adolph Hitler as one example of a charismatic, though evil, individual. Throughout the course of history, there have been many more such examples. But for now, let us return to charisma as a force of good, as something we either have the good fortune to be born with or the intention to obtain, as many components of charisma as possible.

Let us start out with the premise that charisma is magnetism—a form of attraction. Why not then, improve and increase your appeal in every way you can so as to make yourself more attractive? Not in a romantic or sexual sense but in a day-to-day, business sense.

Have Your Colors Done

I look ghastly in pale blue and gray—cyanotic and sick. I knew that before I had my "colors done," but not everyone does. If you want to draw people to you, you have to be attractive—in dress, posture, hairstyle, make-up, or facial hair. Color is important, as are voice quality, words, enunciation, and grammar, and you had better have something important to say in an interesting manner and style. Watch those colloquialisms. Do not say, "havin'" instead of "having," for example, and make an effort to pronounce words correctly. Take an axe to the oft' said I will "axe" you a question. With a lot of practice—and it is worth it—those who were raised with the reverse "s" and "k" sounds can and should place these sounds in proper juxtaposition. You want everyone's attention to be riveted on what you say and not on how you say it.

Study photos or paintings of charismatic individuals you know. Pay particular attention to their eyes and hands. Check to see if they are looking up or down, or at their audience. Are their hands hidden, or spread in front of them in an embracing manner? All of this, and more, counts. Are they smiling? If not, is there a smile in their eyes? Is there inner warmth that shines through?

How do *you* appear to a group? Can you maintain eye contact? What do you do with your hands? Have you been videotaped? As we continue to explore leadership in its many forms and functions, think of yourself and what feels comfortable for you.

Because there are many leadership theories, and they often overlap, let us take them one at a time and start with A.

Attitudinal Leadership Theory

This speaks to the measurement of managers' and leaders' values and feelings. Respect and consideration, development, self-esteem, acknowledgment, and the like, are important in the leader/subordinate relationship, along with initiating and maintaining structure. But sometime, one must question what this means on a nursing unit when it feels like a three-ring circus, and many people are making many demands all at once? When you get home at night and someone asks, "How was your day?" you are inclined to say, "crazy."

But is crazy good or bad? The answer is—it depends. What it means to you has to do with *attitude*. Do you like crazy? Do you have an *aptitude* for turning chaos into calm? To come to a conclusion think of AA, and I do not mean Alcoholics Anonymous. I mean *Attitude/Aptitude*. If you have an *aptitude* for leadership and people respect you and want to take your lead, then turn chaos into calm and move forward into patient-centered care. Your *attitude* should be motivational—your aptitude should be for leadership. Under Attitudinal Leadership Theory you will define relationships, deal with deadlines, understand and oversee tasks, identify lines of responsibility, and clarify roles.

Contingency Theory (Fiedler 1958)

This refers to the leader's ability to lead, plus the behavioral style of choice depending on the subordinate's task and group variables.

Contingency theory, like many others, is good for study in the classroom. But when you are in the cauldron of the busy nursing unit, the hours you have spent in academe should have assisted you to build a solid knowledge base, which should have generated your *Attitude* and *Aptitude*. Now is the time for action, and action is *contingent* on resources and need. This brings us back to my economics professor's remark that the answer to every question and condition is, "it depends!"

The bottom line is that you need to study all leadership styles. Know them all. Know when to apply one and shun the other. Be flexible. Swing with the punches and keep your eye on the goal. Remember what that is? It is ever and always patient-centered care.

Approach that goal with feeling—empathy does not take time, it is an attitude. Apply it across the board. Your staff members—including support staff from all departments—are your emissaries. They collectively spend the most time with your patients. Treat them with care.

Autocratic, Participative, Laissez-Faire—Situational Leadership Styles Hersey and Blanchard (1969)

Situational leadership is my favorite because it fits the leadership style to the individual and the environment. Are you working with a new graduate with limited experience? This is a no brainer. Apply the authoritarian or autocratic leadership style.

Seasoned staff knows what they are doing, so invite them to participate.

Advanced preparation? They could possibly take over completely, with no need for supervision at all. Back off and let them fly. Take a laissez-faire approach. That does not mean pay no attention at all. After all, you are still accountable. But do not hover, and do not sweat the small stuff.

A good manager should be able to be participative in attitude, but authoritarian when necessary. It is also important to back off when appropriate. Think how annoying it is to work under a supervisor who cannot or will not leave you alone to do your work—when you are perfectly capable of doing so; or the opposite may be true—you are left on your own when you could use support. The two preceding examples show this in action. Here are a few more for your consideration.

Transactional leaders are those who identify their followers' needs and provide expected rewards for performance. There is little motivation for employees to reach excellence. They sort of plod along doing as little as possible, knowing the paycheck will be there at the end of the pay period. There is no motivation for them to do better. The self-motivated workers will have long since moved on.

Transformational leaders, on the other hand, are charismatic and intellectually stimulating. They inspire followers to rise above expectations. Generating pride and satisfaction along with enthusiasm and a team spirit, they create a work situation in which a sense of accomplishment and satisfaction permeate the environment. They will rise above their ego needs and head toward self-actualization.

Visionary leaders are future oriented. They always have their eye on tomorrow. The problem with this is they might miss today.

And to these, I would like to add my own category:

Reformational leaders. I believe we need leaders who can reform systems that have failed; leaders who are focused on and able to rehabilitate an unsuccessful workforce. They can apply any and all of the above leadership styles and are skillful detectives. While vetting people and problems, they can build relationships with all levels of personnel. Like a juggler in the big top, they can throw many balls in the air and keep them twirling simultaneously without allowing any of them to crash and burn.

One of the skills all leaders and managers need, on both a practical and theoretical level, is how to motivate staff—especially a reluctant or recalcitrant group of people. We have touched on it, but now it is time to take it apart to see what makes it tick. Recently, I have been told by a number of prominent nurse leaders that RNs seem needier than ever; they seek external rewards and morale building. Their work outcomes appear insufficient to satisfy their ego needs. They just do not seem to obtain satisfaction from intrinsic sources and so look for extrinsic reward systems, which means nothing will ever be enough.

Motivation and Morale—You Cannot Have One Without the Other . . .

Before we move to the theorists, let us start with the word *motivate*. While we are on an *M* word, we will look at *morale*, as well. The question is: are these two issues linked in the workplace?

It is pretty clear that the word motivation has the same root as motor, and motor refers to movement. If one has good motor skills, one moves well. A good motor propels, stimulates, and actuates. A good motivator does the same thing.

When you shop for a car, you look under the hood—at the motor. When you interview a potential staff member, there is no hood under which to look . . . or is there?

First, let us try to define motivation. Is it an internal thing, or is it up to management to motivate workers? We know that management can demotivate workers by being bad managers, but it is too easy to just let the subject drop there. Some people are self-motivated—they are the gung-ho folks who always seem energized—even after putting in several shifts in a row. Then there are those who drag their feet no matter what kind of cheer leaders are running the show. So does motivation equate to energy?

Motivation comes from many sources, starting with our biological needs. You are hungry, so you eat. You feel bowel or bladder pressure, so you go to the bathroom. If you do not meet these needs, over time, there is little else you can think about. A grumbling stomach or a full bowel or bladder pretty much occupies your mind.

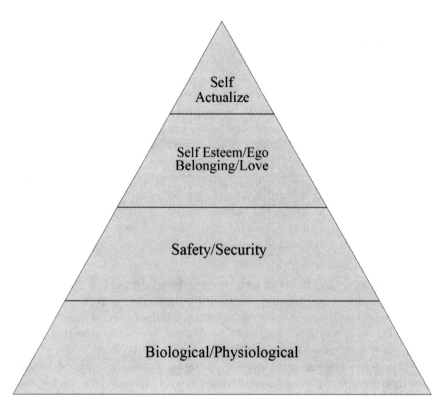

FIGURE 3.1   Abraham Maslow's Hierarchy of Needs. *Source:* Maslow, A. (1970). *Motivation and personality* (2nd Ed.). New York: Harper & Row.

Motivation can also come from an external source, like a sandwich when you are starving. Someone holds it in front of you and says, "Do this "or "do that, and this is yours." If you are hungry enough, you do it. Motivation can come from an economic source—the rent is due, so you work; or it can come from danger—you are trapped in a well or facing a terrible illness, so you pray.

If you are a moral person and you find someone's wallet with ID, you return it. If you are a thief, you know what you do. If there is a meeting of your peers, and the moderator does not show, a good leader walks to the lectern and takes over the session. If you are a follower, you put your head down and become invisible. People who are eager to self-actualize—to advance their knowledge and position—never stop learning.

If you have learned motivation theory in school, you will already have recognized what follows:

The Hierarchy of Needs depicted above is taken from Abraham Maslow's work. It depicts human needs in a sort of a pecking order. Until the first order of needs are satisfied—like hunger and thirst, most human beings can focus little attention on the other needs, like ego fulfillment. So starting at the bottom, we find the physiological and biological needs such as hunger, thirst, clean air, and other basic life requirements. Before most normal human beings can think about fulfilling the next level of need, these must be met. A person who is hungry, thirsty, or freezing cold cannot be expected to think long about mastering complex or even simple human relation issues, or meeting the needs of others.

But once these basic needs are met, we can turn to safety and security needs, all vital components to health care. Strangers wandering through our halls spell danger. Partner this with malfunctioning alarm systems and security guards asleep at the switch, and you may have a formula for disaster.

There also are a myriad of things that only you know about in your facility. These need to be addressed and resolved before you can think about moving up in the ranks to fulfill your social and ego needs to become a leader.

Regarding social needs: even in the workplace, human beings are social creatures. Forget that, and groups of workers will find ways to meet their social needs on company time in ways that do not serve organizational goals.

Go back and read that again and think about how, in the context of effective management leading to patient-centered care, you can provide a social milieu. Remember the mantra: *Empathy doesn't take time.* It takes a caring attitude and approach.

Take a few moments at the start of a shift or the beginning of a meeting to show that you understand this and that you care about your staff members' human needs. Try to remember birthdays and personal and employment anniversaries. Come to meetings with a tasty treat. But most importantly, ask your staff members how they are doing—and listen to their answers.

Once there, you can turn your attention to climbing higher on the pyramid—into the spheres of self-esteem and ego. Here you are seeking fulfillment, achievement, responsibility and meaning. After all, is not that what leadership and management is all about?

Once you feel satisfied at these levels and pursuits, it is on to the top and beyond—on to self-actualization—to be all that you can be, and that is where lifelong learning comes in. A true professional is internally committed to that as an enduring goal. But no matter how high you climb as a nurse leader/manager, the commitment to your staff and patients is always a primary concern.

Vignette   If You Think I Can Help—Ask Me

This is what the assistant director of nursing (ADN) told her staff at a recent around-the-clock meeting. The next day, she arrived at her office to find a NA sitting in the ante room with a teenager sprawled out on a bench next to her. "Help me," beseeched the aide. "You said you would help us."

"This is not what I meant," thought the ADN, as she motioned the aid to follow her into her office.

"They discharged him from the city drug facility and I don't know what to do," said the NA, beginning to cry. "He's been drug-addicted for years and he's only 14. Can you help? Please don't send him back to the city hospital. He has threatened suicide if I take him back there. Please!"

The ADN agreed to help. She picked up the phone and dialed social service. Before the day was out, an inpatient drug treatment center accepted the youngster for care. The ADN's promise—although she had not intended it for personal matters—was fulfilled. Staff-centered care was accomplished. The staff grapevine carried the story, and staff members throughout the facility were rapidly apprised of the outcome. This, in turn, positively boosted morale, thereby constructively affecting patient-centered care.

It is not often that we are called upon to help a staff member get a drug-addicted teen into treatment. But as nurses, we should not turn our backs on those who need help with personal medical issues. Here is another case in point:

Vignette   Look at This

A NA entered the office of a CNE and locked the door. Without explanation, she unbuttoned her uniform top and lifted her bra exposing large, pendulous breasts. She stood squarely in front of her startled CNE and said "Look at this."

The CNE could not help but look, and as she did so she noticed a vast difference in the size of the woman's breasts. She asked her to sit down and requested permission to examine her. In the larger of the two breasts, she palpated an approximately 4-cm mass. The other breast appeared normal.

As gently as she could, she advised the woman that she needed to see a doctor as soon as possible. With her permission, she would set up an immediate appointment with the chief of surgery whom she had seen in conference a few moments ago. The NA agreed.

What is important to this discourse is the level of trust these two leaders had established with their staff members. They had communicated a degree of caring and human concern that may have cost them some time, but also fit into the tenets of the profession they had chosen. It also served their staff members and ultimately their patients in establishing a firm foundation for sustained morale, motivation, and patient-centered care.

As a footnote to the above vignette, the NA had breast cancer and required an immediate mastectomy with follow-up treatment. Had she not trusted her CNE, precious time may have been lost, possibly along with her life.

Motivation and morale are important issues for nurse leaders and managers to bear in mind; there is never enough money in a paycheck or enough time off. Over time, it is the soft incentives that keep a workforce on point—anxious to establish and meet objectives. It is things like humanistic, empathetic, relationships that sometimes make pay issues shrink as motivational factors over time.

Vignette The Power of the Dollar

A consultant was engaged to work with nurses from two separate services that had merged. One was a religious-based organization with a lower pay scale; the other secular, with considerably higher pay rates. Employee satisfaction levels were extremely disparate. The religious-based staff was very satisfied in their work, while the secular staff was not. In addition, neither wished to intermingle, nor did they want to cross-train or be assigned to one another's facility. The cultures were extremely different, and the management/leadership styles were at cross purposes. The consultant had her work cut out.

This example suggests that salary was not a motivational factor for nurses from the religious organization to accept assignments in the secular institution. There was something more important to them than money. As we journey further into the topic of motivation, these things will become clear.

What Beats Money?

The previously mentioned well-known Hawthorne study in the 1920s was conducted by Harvard professor Elton Mayo and his colleagues at a Western Electric plant. Lighting was changed, and production improved. Over time, production declined, so lighting was returned to its former level, and production once again improved. What had been theorized and was substantiated was that human beings need and respond to attention—even negative attention. Many of us have also seen this on our nursing units, not only from staff and physicians, but from patients and visitors. Nobody likes to be ignored.

Once we are aware of these tendencies, we can put them to good use. Like empathy, noticing and rewarding positive behaviors and outcomes rarely takes time. What it takes is sensitivity and good observational skills. People like to be applauded for a job well done.

I remember the story of a NA who was as proud as she could be after giving a patient a satisfying bed bath. She then made up her bed so neatly, you could bounce a dime off the top sheet. Her smile was as broad as all outdoors, as she waited to show off her work. But her supervisor, who was taking a new director on tour of the unit, walked right past her without stopping. The NA slumped in disappointment. She became a negative influence on her unit from that day forward. All it would have taken from the new director was a "well-done" to have kept that NA well-motivated. Instead, she became a distraction.

Alphabet Soup

We have looked at AA for Attitude and Aptitude and CCC for Collaboration, Communication, and Cooperation, and we have examined the GWYNs for Go Where You're Needed. Now we can jump to the end of the alphabet for the X, Y, and Z styles of motivational management.

These will help us understand human behavior in the workplace. According to the work of Douglas McGregor (1960), Theory X individuals—average human beings—inherently do not want to work. They therefore lack ambition, need direction, and require control and force to *make* them do the job. Theory Y people, on the other hand, *like* to work. They therefore will accept responsibility and are self-directed for goals to which they are committed. Praise, respect, and empowerment are more motivating to these employees than are money and benefits.

Imagine what it would be like to work for a Theory X manager if you are a Theory Y employee, or a Theory Y manager if you are a Theory X employee. Remember, Theory X and Theory Y managers each behave toward their employees as if they have the traits they expect them to have, or vice versa.

Also, think about whether or not a Theory X worker can be motivated by a Theory Y manager to shift to Theory Y—a self-motivated worker. Here is a hint: it will take a long time. Trust will have to be developed. Like a rubber band being induced to assume a new shape, slow stretching over time will work better than a sharp tug, which adds to the risk of causing the band—or worker—to snap.

Before we move on to more theorists, let us take a look at nurses on the job and think about what motivates them—or what demotivates them—in the patient care arena. What is it about the patient/nurse relationship that inspires nurses to reach to, and sometimes beyond, their capacities? If we fully understand that, we can translate it to leadership.

A Cry in the Night

Some nurses and their support staff at times turn a deaf ear to a quiet moan or rush past a patient whose face is twisted into a grimace of pain or anguish. One would think that human suffering should arouse them to help, not to rush away no matter how busy they might be. After all, they are caregivers—that is their calling. Students of human history know that in the chronicle of human events, genocide and cruelty are repeated in every generation. There seems to be no end to man's inhumanity to man. But we nurses, in our halls of healing, must not become a part of that—deaf and blind to others' suffering because we are too busy to stop and help.

This does not happen, you say. But I regretfully say it does, and many of the vignettes in this book are examples of all too frequent events reported by patients, physicians, and nurses and other colleagues. As Eli Wiesel, the

Nobel Prize Laureate and concentration camp survivor reminds us, we must neither turn our backs on human suffering nor deny its existence—not if we wish to retain our humanity.

Nurses and especially you, the aspiring nurse manager who will influence so many others, have a lot to do. But ask yourselves as you read: Will that soft moan, that cry in the night, the words "Mama," or "nurse, help me, I'm in pain, I need you," motivate you to step forward? Or will you hurry away because you are so busy with rounds and meetings and countless other things that you simply believe you do not have time to stop?

Will you turn a deaf ear or hardened heart? Think now how each time you do, you might not have another opportunity to help. Patients die, and by extension, not only might your patient suffer and die, but all of humanity—including you—might lose another piece of itself.

Perhaps John Donne, the English/Jacobean poet/preacher, 1572–1631, said it best: "Any man's death diminishes me, because I am involved in mankind: and therefore never send to know for whom the bell tolls: it tolls for thee."

Inspiring a Workforce

We speak of inspiring a workforce, of motivating others to reach for high levels of achievement. But how high can you reach when you are already exhausted? Today's reality is that sometimes those who comprise our health care workforce are already tired because they are employed at more than one job. They may be working three 12-hour shifts in one place and a couple of 8-hour per diem shifts in another. They may also be parents of young children and children of elderly parents. Perhaps they have already put in a shift at home shopping, cooking, doing laundry, and helping with homework. Now, they have to face 8, 10, or 12 hours of hard physical and emotional labor caring for the sick.

There is no more taxing work than nursing—especially when it is applied empathetically. But there is no more satisfying work, either. In that is the motivation to press on. But that does not mean nurse managers cannot learn from other industries. For this, let us turn to a researcher who used a methodology that achieved stunning success.

Theory Z Trumps X and Y

William G. Ouchi wrote *The M-Form Society* in 1982. I use this old reference because if you will remember, that was when the Japanese auto industry pulled ahead of the American auto industry, and we never quite caught up. One of the key reasons had to do with their management style as it compared to ours.

But before I elaborate on Japanese management style, let us take a quick look at General Motors (GM) and its fall from grace. For example, in *The New York Times*, Monday, June 1, 2009, the headline read: *G.M. Heads to Bankruptcy Protection as Government Steps In.* Beneath this headline is a subhead stating: *G.M.'s troubles have hit a low point with its expected bankruptcy, but they have been worsening for years, with many missteps along the way.*

Next is a bar graph entitled: *The Company's U.S. vehicle production.* It is divided into decades, starting with the 1960s and ending in 2008.

- In the 1960s, GM was criticized by Ralph Nader for safety issues. He focused on the Corvair. Instead of fixing the problem, GM hired detectives to investigate Mr. Nader.
- In the 1970s, after the oil crisis, consumers turned to small cars. GM developed the Saturn, but their multiple brands competed with one another.
- In the 1990s, strikes and generous benefits took their toll, and in the midst of the oil crisis and concerns about global warming, the company focused on SUVs and rolled out the gas guzzling Hummer.
- In 2008, GM execs pleaded with the federal government for a bailout, and they had the nerve to fly into Washington, D.C. on their private jet planes! One would think they did not have a clue, and in my opinion, one would be correct.
- As we neared the end of 2009, the individual running GM was removed from his post.

Sometimes looking back makes a picture clearer. But it is hard to fathom how the company, headquartered in a building that looks as solid as steel, shining there at the top of the manufacturing world, could have failed so miserably. GM's leadership had five decades of choices. Yet, it seems that at every fork in the road, they made the wrong ones. We all know that from the results. Like the patient care vignettes throughout this book, I did not have to be there to know that poor care was provided; I only had to know the consequences. What follows is a story that speaks both truth and consequences.

Vignette But He Has Diarrhea. . .

A nurse receives a telephone call from a friend on the opposite coast. He begs her to visit his childhood buddy who is languishing in an ICU across town. "Please," says the friend, "My friend is dying but wants to die at home. He's so very sick; the staff doesn't think he can be discharged. See what you can do."

The nurse travels to the hospital—a large, well-known, university-affiliated, medical center honored with Magnet Status. She enters the ICU waiting room and meets with the wife, who is expecting her. They chat for a while, and the nurse learns that the patient is in an advanced stage of amyloidosis and is receiving hemodialysis three times weekly. They are attempting, with little success, to wean him from tube feeds, which are being given via nasal cannula. Apparently, he is choking on the pureed matzo balls that the wife is adding to homemade chicken soup. The "visiting" nurse counsels against any particulate matter during the weaning period and wonders to herself why staff has not done likewise.

He has a Foley catheter and a rectal bag to catch loose and nearly continuous bowel leakage. He also has a stage five decubitus ulcer that has begun to erode his sacrum and causes him excruciating pain. He is in the end stage of his disease with little time left to live. Both he and his wife want him home.

The nurse enters the ICU cubicle and is overwhelmed by the longing in the man's eyes. He is lucid, friendly, and intelligent. With his permission, she examines his sacral area and is frankly horrified by the extent of the damage. She keeps this to herself. Re-dressing the area, she discusses the risks, benefits, and methodology to getting him home. Having been a home care nurse herself, she believes the plan to take this patient home for the final stage of his life is eminently possible because of his cooperative and capable wife and his deep desire to go home.

With the patient's and wife's permission, she seeks out the primary nurse. This patient, it turns out, is her only patient. This ICU is on a one-to-one patient-to-nurse ratio.

They discuss the situation, and the "visiting" nurse inquires about the decubitus. The nurse responds that the patient has diarrhea. No matter what the visitor says or inquires about, or explains, or expresses doubt about, the nurse repeats and repeats again: "But he has diarrhea." It was as though this explained everything.

When the nurse repeated this story to me, her exasperation knew no bounds. Her voice was tense, her fists were clenched, and her face red.

"What did you say to the ICU nurse?" I asked her.

I said, "But you have only one patient. How could you allow him to develop so terrible a pressure ulcer?"

"But he has diarrhea," the nurse responded.

With hospice and visiting nurse help, this patient was able to go home and spend the final stage of his life surrounded by his family. He did not have to remain in a hospital bed confined to an 8×8-ft cubicle. His loving wife no longer had to strain herself to juggle home responsibilities, a job, travelling to and from the hospital, and cooking for her husband and caring for herself. She finally had him home with her, where their children and lifelong friends could readily share in the life they had led, and now in the impending death made easier by proximity and desire.

Empathy so lacking in the hospital filled this home and strengthened the hearts of everyone concerned. The remaining question is why the nurse, who cared for this once vibrant man, did not understand her role both as a nurse and as a human being. Why did she not know in her nurse's mind and heart that the answer to the question, "How could he have developed so terrible a decubitus while on one-on-one nursing care?" was not, "He has diarrhea." The answer was, "We did not care for him adequately."

Even while he was dying at home with proper care, his pressure ulcer was reduced from a stage five to a stage three.

RES IPSA LOQUITOR

The Fork in the Road

Yogi Berra, the great Yankee baseball player is reputed to have said, "When you come to a fork in the road, take it." The question for you, the nurse leader/nurse manager, is what will you do when you come to a patient care fork in the road? What route will you take? Like General Motors, will you take the path of a monolithic manager and keep yourself away from the fray? Or will you get involved and participate in the action?

Let us look at what the Japanese did to ace American production during the 1970s. There are lessons to be learned and applied to all kinds of management and leadership—especially nursing management and leadership, where our end product is not cars but precious human beings.

Some of the tenets of Japanese leadership germane to American organizations include:

- A consistent philosophy as bedrock to the organization.
- A participative approach to decision making.

■ A holistic concern for people: stable employment and even lifetime employment, whenever possible.

■ Infrequent evaluations and promotions for the first 10 years.

■ Collective values—an attempt to humanize the organization.

■ Structure and incentives.

■ Development of interpersonal skills at all levels.

■ Involve unions—break the rivalry.

■ Egalitarian distribution of power. Again, humanize the organization.

■ Subordinates and superiors become one team and are temporary equals.

■ Trust and support.

■ Enthusiasm at all levels.

■ Common objectives.

■ MBWA—management by walking around. Move the manager's desk to the center of activity.

■ Even the lowest-level employee can stop the assembly line in an urgent situation without supervisors' permission.

Here are two similar U.S. hospital examples. A hospital in North Florida allows all employees to allocate up to $500 to correct a problem without permission. At a South Florida hospital, a five-star program invites anyone to place a star on a bulletin board in the administrator's office for a special service award for an employee who has served above job description. Five stars earn an employee a monetary award.

Earning a Star

She was 85 years of age, arthritic, had osteoporosis, and required a walker. Her daughter-in-law and she went to a five-star hospital to visit her husband (and her companion's dad) who had been admitted the day before for observation and treatment of coronary insufficiency.

The daughter-in-law pulled into a parking spot about 25 yards from the hospital entrance and removed the walker from the backseat of the car, preparing to assist her passenger from the car.

"Wait," called out a groundskeeper. "Wait, I'll get you a wheelchair." And so he did. Not only did he get one, but he assisted the woman into the chair, ensured her comfort, then wheeled the chair into the hospital and up to the unit.

The daughter-in-law asked him his name so she could compliment him to administration.

He asked that she note it on the Five-Star Board and explained to her what it was and where it could be found. She gladly did so.

Applying Theory to Practice

In the classroom, we study many things. We consider leadership's and management's effects and effectiveness, its various styles and applications, what feels right with our personalities, our patient's needs, and our organizational and personal goals and missions. Some of us begin our analysis at the baccalaureate level and then continue through masters and doctoral programs. But when we try to apply those styles that feel best—and that we think best suit the situations we encounter—we find ourselves immersed in the often difficult environment of today's health care culture. Here, there are too many patients and too few resources, interdisciplinary staff that fail to cooperate outside of their disciplines, union workers that are more concerned with protecting their union's turf than with collaborating with non-union staff for the good of the patient, and nurses undercutting doctors who act arrogantly toward them.

Support staff may be working at odds with one another; supervisors sometimes behave like petty dictators or are absentee managers. Chief Nurse Executives may never meet with off-shift staff, or when they do, they are strangers to one another.

The list is long. The pity of it is that most of the participants whose behavior has been reported on these pages have graduate degrees to attest to their education in the leadership and management fields of endeavor.

Here is where reform is needed. And that is why I have dubbed it *reformational leadership*, to be discussed within leadership style context. If we are not honest enough with ourselves to at least admit our shortcomings, how can we fulfill our obligations to those we serve?

If one asks subordinates in a failed system how it *feels* to be in this hierarchy, they report feeling demotivated and dissatisfied. They may appear petulant and uncooperative. It is an every-man-for-himself environment; oppressed group behavior as described by Roberts, exists. Nurses do indeed continue to "eat their young."

A more current reference is by Theresa Brown (2010) who refers to "harsh, sometimes abusive treatment of new nurses . . ." a dirty little secret of nursing. . ." and about senior nurses who lied about her work, refused to help her, and corrected her inevitable mistakes loudly, and whenever possible—publically. Would that these were singular events, but we know they are not. Horizontal violence is extant and trickle down animosity, punishing conduct, and negative social interactions often exist both within and across cultures.

Despite inroads in preceptorship/mentoring programs for new graduates, there still are places that use reverse seniority to make unpopular assignments—including off-shifts. This puts the least prepared nurses and the patients who rely on them for care in danger. From the phenomenological perspective, imagine how it feels to be that new nurse. She has yet to refine her hands-on skills but is placed in a position of hands-on activity. Imagine her working the night shift, on which supervision and mentoring is at a minimum.

Now place yourself in the position of a patient left in the care of that inexperienced, often fearful newly graduated nurse? How might you feel? You would not have been formally introduced to the fact that she was newly graduated or newly employed, but her hesitation would inform you and sometimes she herself would inform you. I have personally heard of new grads who have asked patients to tolerate their clumsiness because they were new. In these cases, the patients invariably reassured the nurses.

Clearly, this practice needs to end. There are solutions. The obvious one is a ubiquitous new graduate preceptorship program. These exist and function extremely well in many large, well-funded medical centers. But in smaller cities, where money is tight, often seniority prevails, so last in means first onto off-shifts.

In an organization with good labor relations, one can work with the union to create a separate category for new grads, to take them out of the seniority line-up for a prolonged orientation/preceptorship period. Union officials do not want untested, untrained nurses caring for their loved ones. Make it personal to make your point. Where there is a will, there is usually a way.

PHENOMENOLOGICAL PRECEPTORSHIP PROGRAMS: WALK A MILE IN MY SHOES

An effective preceptorship program is *not* an extension of an orientation program which familiarizes an employee to policies, the physical plant, mission, vision, and goals of the organization and the like. A preceptorship program *follows* basic orientation.

Many organizations have good preceptorship programs. Here are the basics for a program that has been reported to be effectively in use in Beaufort, South Carolina:

- 12 weeks for new graduates; modified to the needs of experienced nurses.
- Preceptors are selected based on clinical and mentoring skills and their ability to reflect the medical center's vision, mission, and values.
- Once selected, preceptors are enrolled in and must successfully complete an 8-week preceptorship course.
- Before the program begins, both preceptor and potential preceptee complete a Teaching Style Self Assessment Tool to illustrate their particular teaching style. This ensures that the preceptor is able to modify teaching style to the learners' needs.
- During the preceptorship program, weekly evaluation meetings are held between the new nurse, preceptor, clinical instructor, and department director to ensure professional and clinical objectives are met and to allow new nurse to express concerns.
- Patient load is gradually modified and increased.
- Each new nurse is scheduled time to work with the interdisciplinary team appropriate to patients' needs on the unit of assignment.

This appears to be the ideal. Modify it to make it real to your organization.

There are some things that should not be sacrificed. These include the fact that preceptors should be educated in the basics of adult learning, and they should be assigned to the same schedules as the preceptee—on the same unit and shift that the new employee is to work. That new employee should *not* be counted as staff, no matter what. . . If the new employee—professional or support—fails to meet standards, let her go while still on probation. If you do not, you will probably live to regret it—and so will your patients.

One of the greatest morale busters is losing a new nurse, or even a patient because someone—perhaps you—did not properly teach her to crawl before you left her to run a marathon on her own. When someone is brought to the ER with an acute MI or CVA, there is that golden hour—you know that life saving moment in which to act.

This is no less true with a new grad, except you have about 6 weeks during most programs. If you leave her to flounder on her own, you just might ruin or completely lose a nurse forever. Do not let that happen. Not only will patient care suffer, but you will have breached the ethical and moral lines of conduct and will have impinged on everyone's morale.

It is axiomatic that morale will be low where untested, inexperienced nurses are forced to take on assignments for which they are neither prepared nor qualified. Not only will patients be put at risk, but so too will the nurse, the nurse manager, and the nurse educator. Those making such assignments are either deficient in assessment skills and do not realize that they are making the wrong decision, or they lack the moral courage needed to take a stand against such practices.

Here is a story of just such an event:

No One Else to Send

"I won't go," said the experienced nurse with high seniority when called by the staffing manager. "I don't have to go, I'm already settled in and have started my work—and I have the higher seniority."

"But," said the manager, "No one else is available and you must go."

Nurse: "Send Ms. Smith—she's lower on the seniority list."

Manager: "But she's totally inexperienced."

Nurse: "She can do it, and I oriented her yesterday."

Manager: "One day orientation is not enough."

Nurse: "It's enough—I'm not going—you can keep an eye on her."

Manager: "Oh All right."

This manager lacked moral courage and caved. What would you have done? What I would have done is offered her a choice—accept the new assignment or go home with a disciplinary warning.

I know some of you are probably saying, "but then you'd be short another nurse." And I say, "one bad apple contaminates the whole barrel."

Although the next story is not of mis-assigning an unqualified nurse, it does speak of someone *with* the moral courage necessary to take a stand against what she considered to be a miscarriage of justice.

Vignette   She's Just the Gal Who *Could* Say No

In the days of retrospective reimbursement, long before diagnostic-related groups (DRGs), there was a director of nursing at a skilled nursing/rehabilitation facility. She had been with the organization for 9 years, arriving shortly before it opened. The facility was upgrading and accepting patients with a higher level of nursing care needs than previously.

She had worked long and hard on a proposal to increase the numbers of RNs to meet the new nursing care demands. Soon, she and her administrator went to the state capitol where she made her presentation. The fiscal representatives boosted her annual rate by about $350,000. The next day, as she was figuring how many RNs she could add to her staff, her administrator asked her what she was doing. When she told him, he said he was shifting the money to the medical program.

She turned in her resignation the following day.

The above vignette speaks to strength of character and commitment to patients and to self. It also speaks to something more subtle. This individual had strong psychological well-being, confidence in the future, and moral courage, and that, according to many authorities on the subject next to be studied—indicates someone with strong morale.

The meaning of this word, according to Webster's is the level of individual psychological well-being based on such factors as a sense of purpose and confidence in the future, and of course, one can readily see the word *moral* contained within. This refers to right and wrong, or ethical principles, a subject we will cover later, along with critical thinking.

Let us use the previous example—the director who first went to the state capitol and then left her job—to study the principles of right and wrong, plus courage of conviction, character, and common sense.

Surfing the Net for Info

I like surfing the net. The trouble is, it is time consuming and addictive. The good thing about it though is that it can take you out of your specialty—nursing administration—and into something different, such as stock trading. And in this day and age of hedge fund managers making and losing fortunes in seconds, I thought this would be an interesting avenue of study. What constitutes psychological well-being for a stock trader?

According to author Brett Steenbarger (2010), the four pillars of psychological well-being are: joy, affection, contentment, and energy. If we put these into general terms, we can apply them across the board and say that individuals who experience these four mindsets have good levels of psychological well-being.

It is not up to management to see to it that the workforce is psychologically well. It is, however, up to management to identify those employees who are unwell and assist them in obtaining help. To do otherwise is to expose others—both other staff members and patients—to unacceptable and sometimes disruptive behavior. This could adversely affect the morale of those "others," thereby unfavorably influencing the management climate and patient-centered care.

In addition to psychological well-being, healthy morale also requires the following:

- A sense of purpose.
- Confidence in the future.
- Character.
- Courage of conviction.
- Common sense.

The director in the example surely had a demonstrated sense of purpose—a patient-centered sense of purpose. She was alerted to and had agreed to accept patients with a higher level of nursing care needs. Purposefully, she had prepared a fiscal report in the language of accountants and convinced the budget officials of patient requirements. She prevailed. She had confidence in her future ability to provide proper patient-centered care. Her chief executive should have been overjoyed both with her preparation and with her presentation. Instead, he betrayed her. What is worse, he betrayed his own patients. He showed no character.

She was now at a crossroad. Should she continue on in her position, or exercise the courage of her convictions? From the vignette, you know what she did. Ask yourself what you would have done if faced with a similar set of circumstances.

In resigning, she showed courage, character, a sense of purpose, confidence in the future, and common sense. This last parameter may not be as obvious as the others, but it is just as important. Had she retained her position, her CEO would likely repeat his duplicitous behavior in ways she might never know about until it was too late to undo.

Common sense, therefore, dictated that she remove herself before such an event. Also, a moral person cannot in good conscience work for an immoral individual.

THE ROAD TO NURSING MANAGEMENT

In the past, nurse managers became nurse managers by longevity, fiat, and by being liked. If one was around long enough to become familiar to powerful people and a position opened, poof—you were a manager. Now there is a management specialty with education up to and including doctorates to prepare candidates.

Management is a specialty just as complex and demanding as any other. It has a vast body of knowledge and subspecialties. A graduate management degree may subdivide into business, finance, political science, or health care, to name a few, but there are certain core theory courses that run through most. These include communication theory, management, leadership, motivation, organizational behavior, labor relations, change theory, and human diversity; and for nurses, there the clinical areas of study. So there are no ends of learning opportunities.

But what else is needed to make a good manager? As we have discussed before, the human mind cannot just throw up walls around what is bothering it. So psychology and phenomenology are important adjuncts to successful leadership and management.

Successful managers influence their staff over the long run by being empathetic, fair, and even handed; by being effective communicators; by both feeling and showing respect; by never being punitive; by their willingness to help out in a pinch or even when things are going smoothly; by admitting to errors and apologizing when warranted. Successful managers share a hallmark—their staff will pretty much do anything asked of them. They also share behaviors. They address their staff members by name. They know them as human beings with human strengths, frailties, emotions, and needs. They believe and act as though each staff member wants to do a good job. They involve their staff from top to bottom, in creating new models of care, selecting new equipment, designing new nursing units. They abhor pecking orders and favoritism. They are visible and available—when nothing is wrong, as well as when something is wrong. They are experts at MBWA, and they have a big sign on their office door that states their name and that they can be found on the unit. They do not manage by bullying; they manage by helping.

Yet, we know there still are breakdowns, both in the management arenas and at the bedside. Is it because managers have not effectively applied theory to practice? Have they not been mentored? Is the classroom experience so different from the hectic environment of the care delivery setting that theory goes out the window? Does the rush for supplies, equipment, and other essentials supplant the ability to think critically? Is it the difference between management and leadership?

We know that for managers to be effective, it helps for them to have leadership qualities. These qualities can sometimes be taught, but it is best if they are inborn.

Leaders—Born or Made?

The "born leader" theory postulates that successful leaders are born with certain qualities that make them do well. When you look back to the developmental stages of some successful leaders, you likely will find tendencies to volunteer to lead projects or activities and to do things alone when companions are not readily available. You might find some of these individuals sharing a history of walking on the edge of danger and even defeat. They seemed to inherently know they could not succeed if they did not take chances. In fact, many enjoyed the challenge of going into uncharted territories. They found it fun!

You will likely even see it when they were children. Who takes the lead in play? Who is captain of the team? Who chooses individual sports? Who vies to outdo even herself? Usually it is someone with leadership traits—the born leader.

There are even born leaders in the animal kingdom. I remember when my husband and I went to select a new puppy. In the playpen was a fluffy German Shepherd pup that pushed every other puppy out of the way and picked us to be his, instead of the other way around. He was a born leader of dogdom, until the end of his life.

The Born Leader Theory

General Electric CEO Jack Welch is a business author and developer of Six Sigma (a business management strategy that seeks to improve quality). Welch believes that extroverts, with their charisma and "superior verbal skills," are natural leaders. Examples of such leaders are Dr. Phil and Oprah—people who are extroverts by nature and therefore demonstrate leadership qualities like assertiveness, creativity, charisma, public speaking abilities, and style.

From the phenomenological perspective, the effective leader is always *striving to be.* This places the leader in the position of self-examination—one who views personality as distinctive traits that include nature (genetics) and nurture. The author Patrick Chudi Okafor, in his book *Self-Confrontation, Self-Discovery, Self-Authenticity and Leadership* (2009), delves into leadership theory, connecting personality to spirituality, as well as modern leadership theory, motivational theory, and spiritual psychology to enhance issue resolution.

It is the innate leadership qualities that are especially important in difficult and even in dangerous situations, because the leader who has them will likely resolve issues quickly and successfully. Studies are currently being done on genetic similarities of these kinds of leaders—those who are most likely to survive a plane crash, perhaps, or save a life by taking immediate action. What follows is such a story.

Vignette Out of the Mouth of a Babe's New Dad

She was on her lunch break when a man, a visitor in his twenties, got up from an adjacent table and walked toward the door. Although there were no outward signs of trouble, her nursing intuition told her something was wrong. She left her tray on the table and followed him all the way into the men's room. Still, he showed no evidence of distress, but by the time he reached the sink he had turned blue and was clutching his throat. He was a large man. Nevertheless, the diminutive nurse wrapped her arms around him and applied the Heimlich maneuver several times until out of his mouth popped a large chunk of hot dog.

Because of her leadership qualities and her nursing instinct, she stepped forward when others failed to notice an imminent calamity. She saved a new father's life. The nurse was honored for heroism, although she said she did not deserve it. She believed she just was doing her job.

Questions and Points to Ponder
- Have you ever been called upon to react in an emergency, and were you able to take action effectively?
- Would you have followed a stranger into the men's room?
- If an emergency call goes out over a loudspeaker in an airplane or theatre, do you respond?
- If there is a fire in a confined place and emergency personnel give you directions that you consider dangerous, would you follow those directions or break away?
- Are you an introvert or an extrovert? How do you know?
- When you get a hunch, do you pay attention?

What follows is an example of a nurse leader who paid attention to her intuition. By so doing, she helped her agency, her patients, and a new employee.

Vignette   The Intuitive Nurse Leader

She was an assertive individual by nature and an experienced med/surg nurse. With no home care experience other than during her schooling, she applied for a public health nurse/case manager position in a visiting nurse service that had several divisions. The director recognized that this nurse would flourish without close supervision, but would resist efforts to curtail her professional interventions or activities. She would, however, be amenable to a professional reporting relationship. So despite her lack of experience, the director hired her and assigned her to an office with a laissez-faire supervisor. Both the nurse and the agency were satisfied with that evolving relationship, and everyone, especially the patients, benefitted. The nurse remained with the agency for more than 6 years.

LEADERSHIP MANAGEMENT REVIEW

Hersey and Blanchard in their seminal work, *Management of Organizational Behavior*, defined three styles of leadership: Authoritarian or Autocratic, Democratic or Participative, and laissez-faire or noninterventional. In situational leadership, the leader chooses the leadership style, depending on the amount of direction required. For a competent worker, one who demonstrates high levels of emotional maturity, a seasoned situational leader might select a laissez-faire leadership style, in which high relationship-participating and selling trumps delegating and telling as a motivational style.

Expertise weighs heavily in the type and amount of leadership and management required. Apply the wrong type and amount and you risk losing a potentially good employee.

For example, a new nurse in orientation requires close supervision, while an experienced nurse—or should I say a *skillful* nurse, because I suggest experience does not always translate to capability—may require no supervision at all. There are always exceptions. One exception is an emergency, when authorities like police or fire officials take over. But these are rare, so let us look at something less unusual. Here is a situation in which expertise overcame lack of experience.

Vignette   Planting the Plant

A new CNE was brought into an organization in which patient outcome was poor. Pressure ulcers were rampant among the long-term patients and the acute orthopedic patients. Interdisciplinary strife was out of control, with physicians and nurses sniping at each another. Nursing team members were uncooperative, and racial prejudice simmered and sometimes boiled over. Labor management problems created an armed camp.

The new executive was expected to transform the organization into a smooth, patient-centered, community-friendly establishment—one that attracted patients, physicians, nurses, and other quality staff. She was also asked to eliminate the many nursing deficiencies identified by federal, state, and Joint Commission surveyors, and to resolve union issues.

What she had going for her was leadership and management expertise, commitment, energy, good humor, and confidence. She knew that people either liked her or grew to like her, and would want to work with her. She also knew that if necessary, she could let people go.

As she drove to work the first day, she reviewed what her mentor had advised her to do: "Greet your staff and then enter your office. Gently but firmly close the door and position your desk set, calendar, photos of your family and a plant."

"A plant?" she had responded, somewhat nonplussed.

"That's right," her mentor said. "A plant will mark your territory and announce that you are the leader. Then, seat yourself behind your desk and use your intercom to invite your staff into your office, thus establishing your leadership position."

Somewhat uncomfortable, she did as advised. But being an informal person, she started to stammer. So she shed the decorum, came out from behind her desk and greeted each member of her staff individually and warmly. The stammering gave way to smooth conversation in time for bagels and coffee to be brought in by the head of dietary, accompanied by several department heads anxious to meet the new chief of nursing. After all, they had not been able to fill the position for over 2 years.

She then established a schedule of individual meetings with the management staff, made rounds to all the units, and posted notices announcing around-the-clock meetings to which all levels of nursing staff were invited.

At those meetings, in addition to introducing herself and her expectations, which were articulated in patient-centered, staff-focused language, she asked staff members to tell her what they expected of her and what they needed. At first, there was silence, and then, as you read previously, a NA requested a shampoo tray.

This opened the door for an active give-and-take discussion and the time allotted to the meeting flew by. She did not get to know everyone present at those meetings, but everyone present got to know her. It was the first time the staff was able to freely communicate with their director. But all was not well, as she was soon to discover.

Vignette   The Buck Stopped—Where?

Shortly after her arrival, she received a 5 A.M. phone call from an irate attending physician. His patient was a 39-year-old mother of five admitted to the surgical service from the ER, and then transferred to medicine once she was diagnosed with cryptococcyl meningitis. She was dying.

They met shortly at the patient's bedside, in time to accompany her to the ICU just a few hours prior to her death.

Upon investigating, the CNE learned that:

- The 4 P.M. dose of IV antifungal was administered as ordered.
- The 11 P.M. dose was not administered because of equipment breakdown.
- Floor staff had been unable to correct the problem. They called the IV team who tried to adjust the equipment to no avail.
- The supervisor was notified, and the floor staff divorced themselves from the situation.
- The supervisor called the resident physician and made one follow-up phone call. There was no response.
- Despite this, the supervisor took no further action.
- The patient continued to deteriorate, but the nurses did nothing until the attending physician was called in at 5 A.M.
- Later, the CNE met with the supervisor. He confirmed the above account and offered no excuse.
- The CNE met with unit nurses, who believed they had discharged their responsibilities by notifying the supervisor.
- The Director of Medicine met with the Resident Physician, who had worked a double shift and was sleeping when the supervisor called.
- The CNE asked each involved RN to write an educational paper explaining the expected outcome of cryptococcal meningitis in the absence of the prescribed antifungal. They also were asked to research the nurse

practice act for their state, which essentially stated that the RN was accountable for patient outcomes.

Soon, the union representing the nurses for collective bargaining—the SNA—filed a grievance on their behalf. The CNE was appalled that an educational process constructed to not punish, but to enhance professional knowledge and patient safety, would be "grieved." She telephoned the SNA professional practices division chair and "filed a grievance" of her own.

Although the collective bargaining division had no official connection to other divisions of the association, influence was applied, and the grievance was withdrawn. Supervisors counseled the involved nurses regarding correct procedure, and the department of nursing education instructors mentored them in researching and writing a paper about expected patient outcome in cryptococcal meningitis in the absence of antifungals.

I have not ended this vignette with my usual *res ipsa loquitor* because, in this case, I do not believe the thing speaks for itself. These nurses failed to place patient safety first. Their professional obligation was to their patient. As such, they could not discharge that responsibility simply by reporting to another person. What do you suppose made them think they could?

Here are some questions for you to consider before you move on:

■ Do you think they did not know what their professional responsibility was?
■ Were they just plain lazy?
■ How about overworked—was that it?
■ Maybe they had not been properly oriented.
■ Do you know your responsibility under your state's legal definition of nursing?

We could go back to the definition of nursing and ask if they understood that they were responsible for the outcome—assuming they knew what that outcome might be, absent the antifungal. But let us give them an out and ask: What would have made it *okay* for them to walk away?

These are all good questions to think about and discuss in the classroom and with your colleagues. For now, I will give you some hints. Laziness, overwork, lack of orientation and similar excuses are not valid for a professional nurse's lapse when a life is at stake. The only possible acceptable choice is *if* a qualified professional accepts the responsibility and relieves them.

For example, if the supervisor had said, "I've got it, I'll take care of it, don't worry." But even then, if the patient continues to deteriorate and no help arrives, I would hold accountable any licensed nurse who did nothing.

This organization was a laboratory for study and for change. It was large and multicultural, with complex issues. It needed effective leadership, professional management, and cross-cultural communication in an environment in which many non-English languages were first languages. It hosted three strong and sometimes hostile labor unions and was located in a high-crime community. Actually, for active, creative leaders and the right management team, it was a terrific place to be challenged, to learn, to teach, and to have a little fun.

In order to be an effective leader and manager in such an environment, one had to be an excellent communicator and understand both the process and the *gestalt*, or the *complete wholeness*, of effective communication. An effective leader must appreciate that first comes influential, proficient, significant communication because from that, everything else flows.

Here is a quick reference for you about productive management climates developed by Jack R. Gibbs (1961). He is well known for his work with groups and personal and organizational development. Succinctly, he posited that: It is up to management to construct a *productive* employment climate, one that is *supportive* and not destructive. One that is *descriptive* and *problem-oriented* rather than evaluative and controlled. Employees will work to their fullest in a climate that is *spontaneous* instead of tricky, *empathetic* and not neutral. If managers are superior and certain instead of egalitarian and provisional, subordinates will keep their heads down instead of developing into all they can be. They will be demotivated and look to escape from a nonsupportive employment climate. Call outs will increase, and turnover will be high. This will negatively impact on interpersonal satisfaction as well as patient satisfaction. Patient-centered care will not be achieved. It is as simple as that.

Now, let us go over these in a bit more detail:

- *Be supportive and not destructive*—The mantra is Praise Publically; Criticize Privately. The only time or reason to condemn someone publically is to save life or limb. Truthfully, when does that happen? If it were to happen, quietly step in and intervene. A Little Public Praise Goes a Long Way!
- *Be descriptive and problem-oriented rather than evaluative and controlled.* In other words, describe, portray, explain, illustrate, educate. Orient the individual to the problem and how to solve it. Do not evaluate the individual as a failure for having committed a wrong.

- *Be spontaneous instead of tricky.* If you see something you think needs to be corrected—correct it as above. Do not wait to do it at a staff meeting and embarrass everyone. Do not wait 3 months or however long to put it on an annual performance appraisal. Do not wait and jump out from behind a rock, and do it in front of the boss—you know what I mean. Be trustworthy.
- *Be empathetic and not neutral.* I have seen nurse managers stand like statues in front of staff members sobbing as if their hearts would break. Is that you?
- *Do not be superior and certain. Instead, be egalitarian and provisional.* As in the above example, that same type of supervisor is never wrong—could that, too, be you? Often that person has her arms folded across her breasts in a self-protective, cynical posture. Her superior air can be seen and felt across a large room. She does not know the phrases "provided that," or "I could be wrong," or the word "maybe," and she has the power to wither a flower or a new grad from across a room. In my opinion, this is the type of person we could do without in nursing leadership.

SUMMARY

This chapter questions whether management and leadership are different or the same, and responds immediately with the answers:

- Management: leads, organizes, directs and controls a workforce toward organizational goals while.
- Leadership: mobilizes, motivates, liberates, facilitates, releases potential and piques the interest, energy and commitment toward any goals.
- Organization and language skills are important tools of the effective manager/leader.
- Praxis prevails:
  - Take the time to learn the applicable theory
  - Learn to appropriately apply theory to practice
  - Become a role model and mentor staff.
- MBWA: The more outgoing and physically active the manager/leader can be, the more she wanders around. The more she wanders around, the better able she is to observe and become a positive influence on staff.
- Leader behavior style: attitudinal, contingent, situational, transformational, and reformational.
- We look at appearance, posture, charisma, ethos and pathos, communication style, and language skills.

- Motivation and morale as a dyadic relationship.
- Make staff part of the solution—not a part of the problem.
- Make yourself a part of the solution—not a part of the problem.
- Apply the phenomenological perspective—treat people as they need/wish to be treated. Develop your third ear. Listen with your third ear.
- Ask your patients and staff members how it *feels* to be on your unit. Ask yourself how it might *feel* to be on your unit.

CHAPTER ENDNOTES

Brown, T. "When the nurse is a bully." *The New York Times*, February 11, 2010.

Charismatic Leadership Theory. http://business.nmsu.edu/~dboje/teaching/338/charisma.htm (accessed May 25, 2010).

Fiedler F. E. 1958. Leader attitude and group effectiveness. Urbana, IL. U of IL Press. http://en.wikipedia.org/wiki/Fiedler_contingency_model. (accessed July 23, 2010)

Gibbs, J. R. 1961. Defensive communication. *Journal of Communication* 2(3):143.

Hersey, P. & K. H. Blanchard. 1969. Management of organizational Behavior. Englewood Cliffs NJ. Prentice Hall.

Leadership. http://www.nos.org/secpsycour/unit-17.pdf (accessed March 28, 2010).

McGregor, D. 1960. *The human side of enterprise*. New York: McGraw Hill.

Okafor, P. C. 2009. *Self confrontation, self discovery, self authenticity, and leadership: discover who you are and transform the leader in you*. United Kingdom: AuthorHouse.

Ouchi, W. G. 1982. *Theory Z—The M form society*. New York: Avon Books.

Political Leadership Theory. www.muwci.net/history.ppt06politicalleadershiptheory.ppt. (accessed July 22, 2010.)

Praxis Process. http://en.wikipedia.org/wiki/Praxis_(process) (accessed March 18, 2010).

Rao N. Theories of leadership: A brief introduction. http://knol.google.com/k/theories-o-leadership (accessed July 22, 2010)

Roberts, S. J. 1983. Oppressed group behavior: Implications for nursing. *Advances in Nursing Science* 5:21–30.

Steenbarger, B. 2009. *Four pillars of psychological well-being*. http://traderfeed.blogspot.com/2009/05/four-pillars-of-psychological-well.html (accessed March 24, 2010).

4

Labor and Management: Need *Not* Be Adversarial

If you want to see the true measure of a man, watch how he treats his inferiors, not his equals. —*J.K. Rowling*

Section Seven of the National Labor Relations Act (NLRA)—also known as the Taft-Hartley Act (Taft-Hartley Labor Act, 1947)—states that "Employees shall have the right to self-organization, to form, join, or assist labor organizations, to bargain collectively through representatives of their own choosing, and to engage in concerted activities, for the purpose of collective bargaining or other mutual aid or protection." This means that they can belong to labor unions, and if you place your attention on the last four words of the NLRA—*mutual aid or protection*—you will see a structure for adversariality. In fact, a look back at the history of labor unions reveals just that—labor unions were formed to protect workers from unscrupulous bosses' greed, and unfair and often dangerous treatment.

Indeed, there are times when labor/management relationships are adversarial. Job actions like strikes, walkouts, sick-ins, slowdowns, and other efforts to interfere with business operations are probably the most blatant. But there are other more mundane situations during which tension between labor and management becomes evident. These generally include times when workers and their managers disagree about the type or amount of work to be done, pay scales, vacation and sick time, and other conditions of employment. But an overarching issue is not pay and benefits—it is human behavior. It has to do with relationships between and among peers, but most especially between and among labor and management.

Throughout this chapter, you will read about issues of collective bargaining. Pay particular attention to matters of the heart—not love in the romantic sense—but respect, consideration, thoughtfulness, concern, and fairness. Think about how you might maintain a professional attitude when your staff is walking a picket line or serving as a union delegate at a disciplinary hearing. Think about how you might cope with the increasing tensions brewing within a struck organization.

113

Vignette Sometimes, You Want to Smack Someone

Several African American nurses approached me while I was making rounds during a lengthy strike. All employees except RNs (who were represented by another union), therapists, social workers, and management personnel were out on a picket line. After 2 weeks of a contentious job action, everyone was tired and edgy. There was no end in sight.

In addition to acute care patients and an open emergency department, we had about 550 frail long-term patients to care for. We decided to not subject them to the trauma of transfer. With the assistance of several local Yeshivas—Orthodox Jewish Schools—we believed we could provide basic services and keep them safe.

Hardly giving me a chance to ask what was wrong, the nurses told me they had had enough of a 44-year-old abusive long-term patient on their unit. He persisted in calling them vile names.

I asked them to be specific, and they giggled—embarrassed. "How can I help if I don't know the details?" I continued as I accompanied them to their unit.

Finally, one nurse said, "I can't repeat the word he used but it was pretty bad."

More embarrassed giggles echoed behind as we arrived at the patient's bedside. There we were greeted with a tirade from the patient, who looked at me and spewed out some pretty despicable stuff—noting my race incorrectly as black.

I suggested he look carefully at me.

Startled, he stared at me and stated correctly—"Oh, you're not Black, you're White," followed by more nasty epithets.

I told the patient that this time he was accurate, and with an ironic expression on my face, I complimented the staff on excellent reality orientation techniques. Together, we cleaned up the patient and headed for the cafeteria for coffee. There, we chatted about the difficulties in caring dispassionately for someone you want to smack instead.

Professional caregivers may try to rise above a situation in which a patient has little or no control over what he says or does. But being human, they are subject to emotional responses and to exhaustion. For management to ignore this is neither smart nor does it serve the overarching goal of patient-centered care.

As we discussed in Chapter 3—Leadership/Management—the motivational researcher Abraham Maslow illustrated this well. As you will recall, he said that before workers can achieve self-actualization—be all that they *can* be—they first must fulfill lower level needs: food, fresh air, fluids, rest, and even recreation. These are all necessary for human beings to succeed, even during a strike. Nevertheless, some managers—especially in situations like job actions, snow storms, and other emergencies—expect personnel to work without respite. The only purpose this serves is to hasten burnout.

Have you ever heard a nursing staff member say, "I don't even have time to pee?" If you have a formula to safely turn off physiological function, please share it. If you don't, then you must make time for your staff to attend to their biological needs and sometimes even to blow off steam. If you don't, then someone else will, and that someone else just might be a collective bargaining agent. Then you will have more people on the picket line than in-house to worry about. So watch what you do and, especially, what you say. Once the words are out, there is no taking them back. With each retelling, they get more and more distorted.

Vignette   The Damage Was Done

"I'm sorry," repeated the nurse manager, over and over again. She had lost her temper with a subordinate newly-hired RN who had been working her heart out during the strike. She was so exhausted that she had been making one mistake after the other; not major, life-threatening errors, but errors nevertheless—things like giving meds an hour early or an hour late, taking vital signs on patients who did not need them monitored, forgetting to take everything to the lab at one time, thus wasting time.

Normally, the nurse manager held her cool, but she too was worn out, and instead of walking away and then counseling the nurse after she had ensured a rest period for them both, she screamed bloody murder—scaring the poor thing to death and embarrassing them both.

By the time the manager got hold of herself, the new nurse was a bag of rags, crying up a storm, and the manager was a wreck trying to think of a way to control the damage. In truth, it was too late, so she did what she could do—she apologized for her behavior and told the nurse to take a break and get something to eat.

All of this could and should have been avoided. Even a short break replenishes energy and output. Most organizations know that during a strike, it is essential to feed the troops. But food, fluids and bathroom breaks are not the only basic human needs that must be met. Believe it or not, recreational needs also need a little attention, or else staff members do not do well during the long haul. Recreation is easier to deal with than you might think. First, look at the word itself—recreation comes from re-create. So let us recreate the paradigm.

Vignette   Peas Porridge Hot

During my first strike, I can remember going to the cafeteria after about an 8-hour stint subsisting on caffeine and an occasional cracker or donut. I felt depleted in every way. As I approached the food line, I could not believe my eyes. Behind the steam table, I saw the CEO dressed in an apron (covering his trousers and shirt) and a large chef's hat. He was dishing up peas and mashed potatoes. His role had been re-created, thus providing the rest of us some recreation.

Many administrative staff members serve meals during a strike. This, in itself, is pretty funny. To get a kick out of this sort of thing needs you to have a tuned up sense of humor in the first place. Another way to get some mileage out of this is for you—the nurse manager—to convert fun to morale boosting, by personally delivering something to eat—donuts or bagels, or better yet, protein-packed pizza or tuna sandwiches to the units to give your staff a boost when they need it most. But do not forget your off-shift warriors and *your* staff on those picket lines. You read that correctly—*your* staff on those picket lines. I think the thing speaks for itself. These people were your partners in patient care before the strike, and they will be again, when the strike ends.

Questions include: Will they return from the strike with hostility or with trepidation? Will they come back to open arms or to an angry nonunion staff? Will teams re-form stronger than before, or will it take a long time to reconstruct?

The attitudes with which staff return likely depend on how they are treated while they walk those lines, and nonunion staff members who held the fort during the strike—who crossed those lines while perhaps being shouted at—need to be given the opportunity to decompress as well. You have a lot of work to do on both sides of the line. Keep your eye on the goal. Remember—it is always patient-centered care—and you cannot provide it alone.

The question is—can you, the reader, put irritation and anger aside to treat returning union staff with respect and consideration, even during job actions? If you can, you might even find yourself interacting with picketers in unexpected ways.

Vignette **Barnaby Breaches the Barriers**

During my first strike as a chief nurse executive (CNE), I was covering the 12-hour or more day shifts, and my associate director of nursing was covering nights. To deal with her 250-lb Great Dane, Barnaby, she had moved into her fiancée's apartment across the street from the hospital. However, leaving Barnaby alone for 12 hours did the apartment—and Barnaby—no good. Barnaby could not be confined to a small space. He could open doors, raid the refrigerator, rearrange furniture, and accomplish an astounding array of un-dog-like activities.

In order to keep some semblance of order, I had agreed to sleep there. After about 1 hour of fitful sleep, I awakened at about 2 A.M. straddled by this enormous canine dripping drool in my face. No matter what I did, Barnaby would not remove himself from the bed.

Resigned to my fate of a sleepless night, I wriggled out from under Barnaby and put on my clothes. Placing a spiked collar around his neck was no easy task, until I straddled him as I would a horse. Then Barnaby and I opened the door. He galloped from the apartment with me flying behind. My feet barely touched the ground as we made a mad dash across the avenue.

We headed straight for the hospital with Barnaby knowing, as only dogs know, that he was going to see his beloved mistress. As we neared the picket line, it readily gave way. Where huge delivery trucks could not get through, Barnaby and I slipped across like a silk thread through the eye of a needle. As we neared the front door, I called out to security to open the door. Believe me, they could not open the door fast enough to get out of Barnaby's way. We dashed through the entrance and into the arms of my brand new boss who greeted us with a look of shock on his face.

By this time, Barnaby's mistress Suzie—alerted to the commotion—had arrived on the scene to calm Barnaby down. But the damage had already been done. It took me years to overcome the reputation that I was afraid to cross the picket line without the protection of the devil dog from hell.

There are many morals to this story, but the one that stands out is this: we expect our staff to report to duty during all kinds of emergencies—natural and man-made, and sometimes, we even make provisions for child and elder care. But what about our pets?

Questions are easy to ask. Answers are not so easy to formulate but no less important. The time for contingency planning is not during an emergency. It is before the needs arise. In this chapter, the example is a job action—and some staff members literally moved into the hospital for the duration. Administration made provisions for them. Some union-represented employees wanted to move in as well. We advised them to stick with their union.

But for now, we return to the end of the strike. That is the time for labor and management to regroup as partners in patient-centered care. Therefore, the less animosity there is during the strike, the better. Keep it impersonal because that is what it should be. Usually, strikes occur over economic issues and that is not personal. However, it is easy for emotions to run high and for things—and people—to get nasty. Do not give them cause.

YOUR LIPS SAY "YES, YES"—BUT THERE IS "NO, NO" IN YOUR EYES

In a management sense—or in any other sense for that matter—do not say "YES" for effect when you mean "NO," and if you are rushed or otherwise preoccupied, it is better to stay off the units than to make cursory rounds. Other than that, it is essential for the existential, patient-centered nurse leader and nurse manager to be seen and heard and, importantly, to lend a hand regularly during a work stoppage. But being seen even during normal times is not nearly enough.

Tom Peters and Robert Waterman, coauthors of *In Search of Excellence* (2004), addressed the importance of effective managers being out and about among staff. They labeled it MBWA or Management by Wandering Around. This concept appears in previous chapters in this book and is an essential, regular behavior for the effective manager. It does not mean just meandering about, however. It is a focused, dynamic, vigorous, exciting activity that generates a force field. There is a magnetism that attracts and energizes others and that brings optimism into the work area.

This competence is especially important during job actions and other stressful situations. But at all times, it separates the truly great leader/manager from the mediocre. It can create partnerships among managers and staff, whether unionized or not.

To properly perform MBWA, strongly consider adding the no clipboard—or empty hand—rule. This allows the existential manager to always be ready to pitch in and help. It speaks volumes to the onlooker. "My hands are free and I'm ready to help you succeed—or to show you how. Whatever you need, I'm here to assist."

Here is an example.

Vignette   Get the Inspectors Off Our Backs

Federal health inspectors had literally moved into the facility because of the strike, which had already lasted more than 2 weeks.

They made it a point to make daily rounds of the units and interrupt a skeleton staff in their work. So I made it a point to accompany the inspectors on their rounds. This served several purposes—I was able to make patient rounds, visit with staff, interact with the inspectors, and at the same time, I could head off any interference they might inflict on the staff.

One day, while I was talking with some nurses, the agents disappeared. Somewhat stealthily, I looked for them. I found them in a utility room. One of the agents had his pinky finger stuck in a mound of mashed potatoes piled on a paper plate on a patient's lunch tray. One of the Health Department regulations defines food temperature when served to patients.

Struggling to maintain a straight face, I asked if he was testing a new fangled food thermometer. Both inspectors blushed profusely and never again—throughout the duration of the strike—did they leave their assigned office. MBWA had paid off in an unexpected way. But that did not stop me from making my rounds for the duration of the strike and frequently thereafter. One day, I dropped into a unit difficult to contemplate. I call this vignette the Maytag Man.

Vignette   **The Maytag Man**

Very young children, from several months of age to 6 or 7 years old, looked strangely alike. They were not moving or crying or reacting to stimuli. Instead, they were resting eerily quiet in their cribs. They all showed symptoms of the same genetic condition known as Tay-Sachs disease, an affliction that strikes Jewish and other populations. In that neighborhood, it was Ashkenazi/Orthodox Jewish residents. Because they do not believe in the use of birth control or abortion, there was often more than one affected child from the same family. Sometimes, there were two or three. But this was not a sad place because the nursing staff kept hope alive, even though death was inevitable.

They loved these children, and they attended to them with tender loving care and kindness—the kind of TLC that all nurses should provide to their patients if they truly had the heart of a nurse.

As I entered the unit, I asked the staff what I always asked, "What do you need?" Sometimes I am surprised at what I hear, but not as surprised as I was on that occasion. "We need a washer and dryer," was their response.

It seems they did not want to send their precious babies' clothes out to the hospital laundry, nor did they want to continue to waste time hand laundering it themselves. Despite my raised eyebrows, I promised them what they requested and signed the purchase order then and there. I had a bit of a challenge getting it past the purchasing agent, but in the end, I prevailed. A week later—while the strike was still in progress—the Tay-Sachs unit staff was granted their wish.

Once again, the picket line parted when the picketers learned what was on the truck and who it was for, and the union-represented maintenance staff readily stepped across their own picket lines to install the new equipment. You see, on that unit, all staff were patient-centered, union and nonunion personnel were partners, and no one refused to do anything that might benefit those children.

For another change of pace, let us consider an all-RN strike at another facility. The question here is: does strikers' behavior on the picket line reflect the labor/management relationship prior to the strike?

Vignette The 12-Foot Rat

A group of RNs marched to and fro on a picket line in front of their hospital. They brandished their union signs and called out to pass-ersby. To listen to them, one would have thought their management was oppressive and mean. In fact, their director was fair, caring, and supportive. Nevertheless, their union representative brought in a 12-foot air-filled rat and tied it up outside their place of employment. They gave no thought to what *their* patients would think of this as they passed this rat to enter *their* hospital for care. Their behavior was rowdy and unprofessional.

Being a good sport, the director sent out a catered tray of cheese—and coffee—which she personally served to her staff. She felt no ill will against these nurses and welcomed them back into the facility when the strike ended.

Unfortunately, many of the middle managers were not so magnanimous, and several of them held a grudge against the nurses who berated management while on the picket line. Neither the staff RNs nor these managers were able to put their differences aside and focus on their common goal—patient-centered care—once the strike ended. Bad feelings prevailed until a consultant worked with them to reconcile their differences.

This is not unusual in a unionized environment, and it takes a steady hand to work through the tensions that often persist. A patient-centered philosophy and consistent patient-focused language can go a long way to ease tensions that can endure long after a strike has ended.

ALL THINGS START SOMEWHERE

What was the etiology of this tension?

The Wagner Act of 1935 gave employees the right to organize, and the Taft-Hartley Act of 1947 (along with its many revisions) then gave employers rights. There has been something of an adversarial relationship between labor and management ever since. Management is on one side and labor on the other. This is no more apparent than at strikes and at bargaining table sessions where management sits across from its own staff. Sometimes, the separation is so vast, it looks and feels like it might as well be the Gulf of Mexico.

This does not mean, however, that we at the bedside cannot establish a collegial affiliation with our staff and with each other as we focus on our patients. The trick is to create mutually respectful relationships with members of the nursing team and others regardless of their union or nonunion status, educational backgrounds, licensure, training, experience, race, religion, national origin, native language, and so on. Elitism has no place in patient-centered teamwork. Nurses cannot do it alone nor should they try. It is the relationships they build with each other and with members of the other disciplines and support staff that will make or break the care patients receive.

Vignette   Who Owns The Operation?

She was the organization's newly appointed CNE. A strong union represented all entry level staff, LPNs, social workers, and office workers. Delegates were militant and did not limit themselves to representing workers from their own departments at disciplinary actions. Managers had received no training in contract interpretation or grievance and discipline procedures. They often said "the union won't let us do that," or expressed similar sentiments.

One of the union vice presidents was known to be a skillful rabble rouser who could rile up a crowd of employees and turn them into an uncontrollable mob. His language was "of the streets," and once he got started, there was no stopping him.

The new CNE was well schooled in labor relations, had a master's degree in health care administration, and had been through a labor action or two. Importantly, she was not afraid to take on the difficult challenges presented to her.

Shortly after her arrival, she was visited by several delegates who wanted to meet with her to explain "how things worked." She refused to see them without an appointment. They milled around for a while, and she called security, as well as their department heads. They returned to their duty stations.

Soon, she was called upon to hear a third step grievance. They all showed up again and started shouting. She called security. After several more attempts, they got the point and made an appointment—one at a time.

Soon the nursing delegate asked for an appointment and requested a transfer to the ICU. Barely able to contain herself, the

CNE reminded her that she had made herself pretty unpopular with her aggressive behavior. The NA—Millie—promised to stay out of trouble, keep the other delegates in line, and do a great job. Now, all the CNE had to do was to convince the ICU nurses.

Although the RNs were reluctant to have anyone other than RNs in the unit, the CNE wanted to try a pilot program with a tech in the ICU to relieve RNs of routine tasks. Opportunity might be knocking. Convincing the nurses to accept this particular individual would be a major challenge.

The CNE met with the ICU staff to discuss the issue. After calming them down, a deal was struck. Since it would be a new position at a new salary, the union would have to agree. The arrangement included the following: Millie would be trained as a nursing tech. Representative ICU RNs would review and validate her skill set. She would be re-certified in nursing tech skills and would learn to work around ventilators.

It would be up to Millie to negotiate with her union to get them to approve the upgrade and to concur with the pay scale already agreed to by Millie and the CNE. If the union tried to parley more or in any way gave management a problem, the deal was dead. This was nonnegotiable. During a 6-month trial period and thereafter, Millie would attend to her union delegate's duties on scheduled time only if and when the unit could spare her.

What started as an experiment turned out to be a roaring success. Millie sported an embroidered shoulder patch announcing her new status: "ICU TECH." She stayed out of trouble and became a role model for other delegates to also behave properly. The CCU and ER soon wanted a tech for their units. A more patient-centered relationship developed within the organization. Union/management interactions remained adversarial, but good nature sometimes snuck in, and patient-centered language started to replace the I's, the me's, and the whining.

Several lessons were learned or reinforced from this experiment, and advances were made:

- Human beings crave attention. If they cannot get positive attention, they will seek negative attention.
- Management must impose limits on negative behavior and maintain a patient-centered approach.

- Union contracts were made available to management personnel, and instruction on interpretation of its clauses was scheduled.
- An "alarm system" was established for a manager to obtain assistance in the event union delegates, officers, or others threatened them in any way or disrupted the patient care environment.

Management operates the patient care/employment environment. Management has rights. Among them are the rights to hire, fire, and discipline. And its management that writes the paychecks.

"UNIONS DON'T MAKE UNIONS—BAD MANAGEMENT MAKES UNIONS"

There was a time—and this is still true—during which some RNs believed that belonging to a labor union was unprofessional. But today, many professionals belong to labor unions. Why do you suppose that is? For the purposes of this book, let us look at RNs.

RNs join unions for the same reasons most people join unions. They believe that collective representation makes them stronger *against* management than they would be as individuals. Unions give them protection in opposition to *unscrupulous employers*. The question is why would nurses need protection from their employers?

Were not questions like these more applicable to sweatshops? In those circumstances, women and children were practically chained to their sewing machines, and many died in fires or of premature old age, disease, or overwork. But nurses do not have to look at sweatshops to seek out examples of being taken advantage of by a system that had the potential to burn them out. Just think about the apprenticeship structure many of us considered normal as our educational process. We worked a full workweek and went to school, as well, and we were paid the sum of less than $20 per month plus room, board, uniforms, and medical care.

This was acceptable only until other opportunities became readily available to women. After that, some who would be nurses sought out other education and employment avenues. These included medicine and law, business and architecture, and other heretofore and still-often male-dominated professions. Irrevocable shortages of registered nurses occurred and created what seems to be an irreversible economic crisis. Nurses—no matter how well educated and essential they are to society—are paid less than male-dominated professions. Additionally, we have yet to solve our internal entry level associate degree vs baccalaureate degree dispute.

I might add, we nurses made way for physicians' assistants, a subject I will cover more fully in the epilogue.

We continue to have a shortfall of RNs and a nursing faculty shortage—especially young, doctorally-prepared educators. To compound this problem, our society is older and therefore prone to chronic illnesses, including cancer and neurological diseases. We are more transient, more vulnerable to attack, and more in need of professional, high-quality nursing care. If staff members cannot rely on their employment organization and its leaders to give them a fair shake, they will seek shelter elsewhere. If they can, they will turn toward a union, and management will have a partner it does not want.

The point is that unions do not create the need for unions; it is generally ineffective or oppressive management that causes staff members to seek protection and representation. They simply do not trust their leaders/managers—and sometimes with good reason.

Consider some of these typical work-related issues:

- Baccalaureate-prepared RNs (RN/BSNs) transport patients because administration will not approve budget for transporters. "Let the nurses do it," they say.
- RN/BSNs make beds because there is no budget for off-shift housekeeping staff.
- "Are OR Techs employed because they are less expensive than RNs?"
- Who obtains stat drugs from the pharmacy? What about stat supplies?
- Who answers phones when unit clerks are at a meal break, or coffee break, or . . .? What about off shift?
- Do managers call upon staff to float long after the start of shift? What is their communication style?

If management will not or cannot solve your issues and your colleague's spouse, partner, or friend is a union member, might you not be coaxed into going to a kaffee klatch—to just at least listen and learn, and once there, might you not *just* agree to sign a card *just* to indicate your interest in learning more?

If enough cards are signed, an election might be approved by the National Labor Relations Board (NLRB)—and who knows where that might lead?

If you are or aspire to be a nurse manager or leader—then you are the one who needs to know. If your goal is management—union or no union—your partners are twofold: your patients, who always come first, and your staff.

Union-Organizing Campaign (Forman & Davis, *JONA*, September, 2002)

Here is the typical scenario that unfolds during a unionization attempt:

■ Employees seek union representation because of dissatisfaction with management.
■ Union representatives will assess the situation to ascertain chances of success.
■ Employees who contacted the union will become the union's representatives within the employment setting.
■ The union will try to keep the campaign secret for as long as possible to encourage anger, wear away trust in the employer, and become confident that the union can fix things.

During this time, it is essential for the employer to become sensitive to signs and symptoms of unrest. Watch for such things as employees meeting furtively in hallways, a chill in the air, sneaky looks, failure to make eye contact, notices posted requesting email addresses, and the rumor mill running at high speed.

The law requires that at least 30% of eligible employees show interest by signing a petition or an authorization card. Most unions, however, will await a 65% to 70% show of interest before filing with the Labor Board. Once this happens, The NLRB will call for a secret ballot election in 42 days.

Management is likely to run a counter campaign to try to convince employees why they are better off without a union. This will only be effective if the facts support the claims. But often it is too late. Think about why employees sought out a union in the first place.

What May Management Legally Do?

■ Management may speak to its employees, but it may not *Threaten*, *Interrogate*, *Promise*, or *Spy*—use the acronym *TIPS* to jog your memory.
■ Management may present facts.

- If the issue proceeds to an election and employees vote to have a union represent them, the union and management then negotiate across a bargaining table with a list of demands.
- The law does not require the parties to reach agreement, only that they bargain in *good faith.*

What follows is an account of a negotiation during which the bargaining committee put forth a demand that could—in the opinion of their director—moderate their professionalism and diminish her campaign to elevate nursing's standing in the interdisciplinary community.

Vignette We Demand Reeboks

The union presented management with a long list of demands. Few were mandatory subjects of collective bargaining, which includes salary, benefits, and conditions of employment.

In an effort to comply with some of them, its representatives considered the list very carefully. Most were frivolous in the extreme, but one stood out as particularly antithetical to the director's goal for professionalization of the staff. The demand was to allow the nurses to wear Reebok sneakers to work. This was long before dress codes were relaxed, allowing all forms of footwear, including sneakers of choice. The management negotiator asked if another brand would do. The union negotiator said "no—only Reeboks."

In an effort to bargain in good faith, the hospital negotiator mentioned several other sneaker brands. The union negotiator was unmoved.

This went on for a while until the hospital negotiator said that he would get back to the union at the next session. Then, the CNE presented a ream of nursing leadership literature tying professionalism and power into appearance. Once again, the union-negotiating committee was unmoved.

Finally, the hospital decided it was not a strike issue and refused the demand. It allowed instead a request for a uniform committee to decide on a change in the uniform code minus a change in footwear.

As previously stated, according to the NLRA, *mandatory* subjects for collective bargaining include salary, benefits, and other conditions of employment. Everything else on the list of demands is discretionary. However, management reps should be cautious about what they accept and what they decline. A majority of their staff has elected for the union to represent them. This should be seriously considered when deciding what to disallow.

If agreement is not reached and an impasse seems endless, the employer can put into effect the proposals it made to the union—without the union's consent. It has the sole opportunity to show its employees willingness to mend relationships. Also, it needs to maintain parity in salary and benefits within the community or it will no longer be competitive.

But sometimes, it is not necessary to walk away from the table. Sometimes, the pathway to a contract settlement comes from an unexpected place.

Vignette   A Voice from the Great Beyond

Negotiations between a nurses, union and a hospital negotiating team had been going on for days. Everyone was worn out. All issues except salary had been resolved. Word had come from an unexpected source that the nurses' union was getting ready to settle for less than the hospital was willing to pay—and about a full percentage point less than was being paid to RNs at a competing medical center in an adjacent community.

The hospital's chief negotiator called a caucus just as the union negotiator was about to put his offer on the table. Everyone stretched, and the union negotiator got up and headed for the men's room. Soon, the hospital negotiator followed.

When everyone returned, negotiations picked up where they left off, except that the union negotiator demanded the higher rate—the one the hospital needed to keep it competitive. After feigned histrionics, they settled. Later, over a drink or two, the union negotiator related a story that he had heard a disembodied voice in the men's room saying: "Don't settle for less than six percent."

For the reader who is scratching her head in consternation, the hospital negotiator had followed the union's rep into the men's room. He entered an adjacent stall. Not identifying himself, he intoned seven vital, enigmatic words that served both labor and management. The nurses got what they wanted, and the hospital remained viable in the marketplace.

Decertification (Forman & Krauss, *JONA*, June, 2003)

Once a union is in, it is in, unless the staff it represents decides to decertify the union or certain groups—bargaining units—within the union. This happens rarely. Nevertheless, it can occur by a process called decertification, which we will discuss regarding a group of supervisors. In comparison to an entire bargaining unit, that process is relatively simple.

Decertification options were established in 1947 with passage of the Taft-Hartley Act or NLRA. Provisions for this process are similar to those certifying a union. Employees wanting to decertify must show that at least 30% of affected employees stand with them. The employer may not promote the process but may, if asked, give information about their rights under the NLRA. The process for decertification is similar to that of certification. But in the case of decertification, the union is not involved.

Once the union has gathered signed cards from 30% of eligible employees, it forwards that information to the NLRB, which calls for an election in 42 days. There are certain protections for a new union, however, and in fact, there are more certification elections than decertification elections.

As in all management environments—it is up to the existential, patient-centered manager to remember and act upon certain givens:

- Unionized employees are *not* the enemy. In your effort to decertify their union status, learn what it is like to walk a mile in their shoes.
- Remember that lack of job satisfaction is a leading cause for employees having sought a union in the first place. What have you done to change that?
- Unions represent employees for collective bargaining. Be sure your employees understand that you represent their best interests.
- Have you opened lines of communication? If you do not, the union will.
- Do not allow the union to comanage operations. Know the management rights clause of your collective bargaining agreement. Apply it with grace and empathy.
- Give your employees reasons to trust and support management. Do not give them cause to continue to seek union protection.

Keep the Momentum Going

Your staff has shown trust in you—they have given you a gift. They have filed for decertification (or you have filed for a unit clarification within your organization. This means you believe certain unionized employees fit the definition of supervisors under the NLRA definition). Do not waste trust. Be sure to make good on all your promises, or the union they decertified will be back with a vengeance. Now, you will deserve everything you will get.

What Happens Once a Union Is In?

The fact that a union has won an election likely means that management has not done a good job demonstrating to staff that they do not need a collective agent to represent them. It does not mean, however, that management must throw in the towel.

Management hires and fires staff, pays the bills, and distributes the paychecks. Management retains the right to direct and control the workforce unless it gives up those rights through inept management or at the bargaining table. These rights include the right to hire, fire, promote, assign, transfer, schedule, layoff, and discipline employees. Management is ultimately responsible for the care provided to *its* patients. In order to best do this, management must work in partnership with the union that represents managements' staff *for collective bargaining*.

That said, there are times disagreements will take place, and role conflict will prevail. In my first job as director of nursing, every RN, including 23 supervisors, were represented for collective bargaining by the same union. The only RNs excluded from representation were three assistant directors of nursing and of course, me. In other words, the nurses these supervisors directed and controlled—management activities—were sisters in the same union (or professional association), its preferred nomenclature.

In order to file a unit clarification (UC) with the NLRB, to decertify supervisors from the union, management would have to provide proof that they spent a lion's share of their time in what are known as *statutory supervisory responsibilities*. Briefly, this means "having authority, in the interest of the employer, to hire, transfer, suspend, lay off, recall, promote, discharge, assign, reward, or discipline other employees; or responsibly to direct them, or to adjust their grievances, or effectively to recommend such action. These supervisors were responsible for directing, controlling, and disciplining their sister union members. This begged the question—

did they perceive themselves to be management first or union members who were expected to stand up for fellow union members? Role conflict was evident, and it interfered with proper labor/management relations and patient-centered care.

We in hospital administration—with the advice of the hospital attorney who also was the chief negotiator—decided to file a UC in an effort to decertify these supervisors. We would have to provide hard evidence to the NLRB that they all fit the definition of supervisor under the NLRA as described above.

These supervisors were responsible for directing, controlling, and disciplining their fellow union members. Where was their allegiance? Was it to management, who provided their paycheck, or to the union and to their union sisters and brothers, which contributed toward a sense of camaraderie? It was my job to shift loyalties—to our patients.

Vignette A Your Name Is Alison; B Your Name Is Bernadette. . .

The hospital attorney advised me that despite my short period of employment—3 months—I needed to know all 23 supervisors by name, shift, and area of assignment. After all, I was the primary witness. Adapting the old song *A—You're Adorable, B—You're so Beautiful . . .* I managed to memorize the 23 names. Adding shifts and areas of assignment came as a tag-on because I had spent many hours with these individuals and had established mutually respectful relationships with them. But now and in this regard, we were adversaries. I wanted to decertify their union status because I firmly believed they were managers, and I felt they needed to be relieved of role conflict inherent in their dual status.

They, on the other hand, had learned to distrust previous management and did not know me well enough to trust me. However, they were also uncomfortable with the conflict, so I maintained a patient-centered approach, using patient-centered language.

While this case was proceeding, the union representing the rest of the staff was making inroads in acquiring signatures from staff nurses indicating their interest in shifting from their existing union to the union representing the rest of the staff if contract negotiations did not resume soon.

But the nurses' union was stalling to pressure the hospital to settle the UC. Neither option was in the hospital's—nor our patients'—best interests. We needed the supervisors decertified, and we did not need all our staff in one union. The nurses' union would share that latter goal.

To accomplish this rather complex series of objectives, I stepped outside acceptable conduct and contacted the nurses' union president. I urged her to meet me in a neutral location to find a solution acceptable to us both. In truth, this was not entirely "kosher." Management and labor should not meet behind the scenes, but in this case, the greater good—patient-centered care—would be served. As with King Solomon, we settled on splitting the "baby"—decertifying some of the supervisors. I would not, however, agree to leave job descriptions untouched. My plan was to make them clearly nonunion for the remaining supervisors—over time.

Since this was an off-the-table meeting, we shook hands to seal the deal, and we each returned to our offices. Sometimes, going around the table is better than staying on it.

"The Union Won't Let Us Do It"

The result was we had a group of nonunion supervisors who understood their rights as managers—correct? Then why would a group of managers in a nearby facility allow a staff of nursing assistants to clock in, then leave to park their cars, or go home to take their kids to school? Sometimes, they were gone for 15 to 45 minutes after their shift began—sometimes longer.

The consultant who was brought in to work with the management team was told two things in response to the same query—she asked them why they allowed such egregious behavior to occur.

Their response?

"That's the way it's always been,"

and,

"The union won't allow us to change it."

These managers had no training in contract interpretation and implementation. In fact, none had even seen a contract—so that is where the consultant began. She also worked with the directors who engaged her services, and she established a meeting with the HR director to ensure support from above. This was long-standing behavior. In order to break it, administrative support was essential. A united front with advance notice to union officials would have to precede any unit by unit action.

Once this was accomplished, employees would be given advance notice of their new policy and that disciplinary action, up to and including termination of employment, would result from noncompliance. They would need to make child care arrangements. An implementation date would be set several weeks into the future and adhered to.

Everyone was advised to be patient, patient-centered, and persistent. As actor John Belushi is reputed to have said: *Persistence Overcomes Resistance.* These managers had allowed this behavior for a very long time. They also needed to take the time to change the paradigm that they created. Ultimately and inevitably, discipline would likely have to be imposed. With that as a backdrop, let us segue into proper discipline use and the disciplinary process.

CRIME AND PUNISHMENT

The New York Daily News contained the following headlines on July 26, 2009:

> *Faked records and fatal blunders at city run medical centers; The cover-ups hid a trail of human suffering among patients who were maimed; A stroke victim's leg had to be amputated after gangrene was left untreated; Logs for a respirator were changed after a staff member noticed it wasn't turned on and the patient died.*

A nurse manager knew what was transpiring and did nothing to correct the situation. The paper promised there would be more examples to come every day for a week. There were.

Short staffing is not an excuse. Lack of concern is not an excuse. Lack of coordination is not an excuse. Frankly, there are no excuses. People lost their lives, and in other contexts, it might be called murder or manslaughter. But to call it health care or any other kind of care is an egregious misuse of the English language.

These are extreme cases and they require extreme action. But in the everyday life of patient activities—and employees—things go wrong, and one of management's more difficult responsibilities is to be able to correct errant behavior with timeliness, finesse, and consideration both for the patient and for the employee.

Formality Pays Off (Forman & Merrick, *JONA*, February, 2003)

Disciplinary action needs to be appropriate, prearranged, standardized, well planned, and authorized. It sends the message that management means business and that transformation is required, or there will be penalties. It also generates a record that can be used later, if necessary, to allow you to progress to more severe steps if the employee fails to correct unacceptable behavior. Lastly, it provides the employee verification that she or he has been treated fairly and according to policy for appeal to upper management, human resources, or outside agencies.

Remedy Does Not Penalize—Unless

It is important that corrective action fits the offense. Minor offenses, such as lateness or dress code violations, may be dealt with through coaching or counseling. Major wrongdoings such as fighting or carrying a weapon to work might call for suspension or immediate discharge. Also remember that:

- Rules should be known. Do not allow ignorance to be a defense. For example, rules in the event of a fire should be in-serviced and posted. Cursing, patient abuse, carrying or brandishing a weapon is universally unacceptable.
- Corrective action should come as no surprise. Managers must be careful to not allow personal bias to influence them.
- Steps of discipline should be progressive. For example, a first offense might result in an oral warning. For the next infraction—a written warning; for the next—suspension without pay; and finally—discharge. More serious wrongdoings might start with more severe penalties, thus eliminating oral and first written warning. Some discretion is okay, but beware even of the appearance of favoritism.

Vignette   Taking a Bite Out of Crime—Or Not

A CNE was performing MBWA when she heard a commotion. As she looked into a patient's room, she observed an NA lean over and bite an elderly patient on her shoulder. As the CNE rushed into the room, the patient cried out in pain, and the NA jumped away from the patient, startled and defensive. The CNE told the NA to go directly to her office and wait there while she comforted and examined the patient. A dark bruise was developing on the patient's shoulder. The CNE pressed the patient's call button and asked an

RN to bring her a cold pack and take over the patient's care. She then called security to photograph the injury and complete an incident report.

After seeing to the patient's safety, she went to her office and advised the CNA to contact her delegate. Once the delegate arrived, because of the egregious nature of the violation, she suspended the CNA without pay pending further investigation and possible termination of employment.

That is indeed what took place—until the union vice president went to the corporate vice president of the health care organization and made a "deal." They agreed to have the CNA reinstated over the vociferous objection of the CNE. They placed her in building services but in the same facility in which she had bitten the patient.

The CNE objected and threatened to go to the health department. She was given the choice of buckling under and accepting the arrangement or resigning. She resigned. Some things *are* worth fighting over.

THE POWER OF THE PEN—OR THE PC

Remember that words can come back to haunt you. Each organization should have a formal disciplinary policy, procedure, and report form. If your organization lacks these things, do it yourself. Be formal in all you do in this important area. Otherwise, what you do or what you neglect to do can cause you and your organization trouble.

You might start with an oral warning—be kind and considerate in tone and demeanor—but be specific and patient-centered. You do not have to be mean to mean what you say.

Make it clear that whatever the offense, it is unacceptable and must be eliminated, or consequences—including further disciplinary counseling, which might include suspension or termination of employment—will follow. What you should not do is what parents often do: "Johnny, if you do that again I will kill you!" Johnny quickly learns that mommy will not kill him, so he does it again and again. So whatever you say you are going to do, be prepared to do it.

If your employee repeats unacceptable behavior, write him up—clearly and specifically. Give the history. Indicate when the oral warning was issued. The question is: should it count, or should you start fresh?

Remember my economics professor's answer: it depends. It depends on the infraction and the circumstances. A constant is that you should always apply rules of reasonableness and your organization's policies and procedures.

But let us suppose the infraction was last month, and it was serious enough to require follow-up. Now is the time for a first written warning. Be sure to include the caveat that suspension will follow the next violation. If the employee fails to improve, the manager should suspend the employee as indicated. In addition, the employee should be advised that termination of employment will follow repeat incidents.

Some organizations have a menu of progressive disciplinary actions— so many days suspensions for a first offense; so many for a second, then termination of employment. Remember, arbitration is the final step in the disciplinary process. The arbitrator will look for written evidence that progressive disciplinary action was taken and that the employee was warned of consequences—specifically warned.

At the point of termination, the effective existential manager should be able to rest assured that she has done everything possible to help the employee understand what lies ahead for failure to correct unacceptable behavior. *Reminder: Being overly kind to an employee may be overly unkind to your patients.*

REPRESENTATION—UNION AND OTHERWISE

Union employees are entitled to representation by virtue of contractual agreements. Most contracts have language that allows for a delegate to be with an employee at any meeting that has the *potential* to result in disciplinary action.

This does not mean they may have an army of delegates accompany them, as has happened in some union settings. When this occurs, it is up to management to put a stop to this behavior. A Machiavellian way is to grant no favor to an employee who arrives in a manager's office with a cadre of demanding union delegates.

A more delicate way is to develop relationships with some cooperative delegates and advise them of the proper approach. Then, allow them to put an end to unacceptable tactics.

Both methods have merit. As to when to apply which? "It depends." What you should not do is allow unacceptable practices to continue without taking appropriate action. Patient-centered care will be sorely interrupted by groups of staff members leaving their posts to intimidate managers who are counseling employees on breached hospital policy.

But what about nonunion employees? Known as *Weingarten Rights*, these are derived from a 1975 Supreme Court case, NLRB vs Weingarten, where the Court announced that unionized employees have the right to representation during certain investigatory proceedings. In July, 2000, these rights were extended to nonunion employees—if they asked for such representation. However, in 2004, during the Bush years, the NLRB reversed itself, holding that Weingarten Rights held only to unionized employees. As I write this, President Obama just appointed a strong labor-oriented individual to the NLRB; so by the time you read this, it may yet change or has changed again.

Before we move on to grievances—the counterpart to discipline—let us look at the topic of anecdotal notes. All good managers should keep a diary of informal conversations with staff noting dates, and both complimentary and critical remarks made throughout a year's time. Commentary about staff members by interdisciplinary personnel, patients, and visitors, should be noted as well.

Other information such as equipment or needed repairs, patient requests, creative ideas, and the like should be jotted down and crossed out when completed. These anecdotal notes should be kept personal and private and referred to when creating performance appraisals, special mention, and disciplinary reports.

These are important because without them only the past several weeks are referenced when preparing annual evaluations. With them, you can access an entire year without being a memory expert. The reason for privacy is so you can write away without concern that someone will have access to your innermost thoughts, and what is not known cannot come back to haunt you.

PERFECTION: THE UNREACHABLE GOAL

Just as beauty is in the eye of the beholder, so too is perfection. Therefore, even when the most experienced, existential, patient-centered nurse manager honestly believes that she has made her schedules and assignments in the most even-handed ways possible, one or more of her staff members might disagree. The next thing the nurse manager knows is that she is presented with an informal or even a formal complaint. In a unionized setting this is known as a grievance.

When this happens there are steps to follow. Let us start with the easy ones first and work up to the more difficult.

- The sit-down: this goes along with the *KISS* rule—*keep it simple, stupid*— or if you prefer—*sweetie*. Have an informal sit-down with the complainer and drink a cup of coffee—or tea, or whatever. Ask what is wrong. Listen carefully. Ask the journalistic questions: Who, What, When, Where, Why, and How. Be prepared to change your mind. If neither of you can convince the other, move on to step two.
- This is a formal step whereby the employee completes a formal grievance report that goes to her manager. This is spelled out in the union contract. In a nonunion facility, it should be in the personnel policy manual.
- If the issue is not resolved at this level, it might go to the department head and then to arbitration, depending on contractual agreements or, it may go to human resources before arbitration, which is usually binding.

In some organizations, in which state nurses associations represent nurses for collective bargaining, the nurses may have been advised to make claims of unsafe staffing based on staff/patient ratios. In these instances, work with your nurses to determine what acuity standards they are using to measure their claims against. It is likely that they are using raw numbers. This gives management a teaching opportunity to include patient acuity in their calculations. Be careful to not make it adversarial.

UNION–MANAGEMENT COOPERATION (FORMAN & POWELL, *JONA*, DECEMBER, 2003)

Lest you think I have written an oxymoron, please think again. Although there is much union/management dissent, it is possible to achieve union/ management cooperation. Think back to the organization at which the union displayed a 12-foot rat near an RN picket line during a contentious strike. At that same facility, not too long after that strike ended, a series of seminars was conducted periodically throughout a year. They covered such topics as effective communication, motivation, 360° customer satisfaction, labor relations, patient-oriented care, conflict resolution, leadership and management effectiveness, and team building.

The management level courses were mandatory for all nurse managers and the nonmanagement level classes voluntary for staff nurses and support personnel. It was then decided to bring all levels of RN licensed personnel together to focus on patient-centered care. For the first time in the organization's history, the union business agent—someone with a reputation for being militant and difficult—was invited to join the group. Staff nurses, who were also union delegates, were to "keep her in line" and focused on patient-centered care. It was broadcast that anyone who strayed from this topic would be asked to leave the seminar.

The meeting proceeded without a hitch, and much was accomplished. Union issues and status never came up—except when the business agent indicated that because *her* delegates were there, she *had* to be there too. Although this comment was ignored at the time it was made, there was a strong rejoinder afterward reminding her that management had the exclusive right to meet with its employees without notifying the business agent or having her present, except as stipulated in the contract. She was welcome to the aforementioned meeting as a guest and at the whim and will of management.

This reminds us of two things:

- Do not allow the union to comanage.
- Mutual cooperation in patient-care matters is key to effective patient-centered care.

If these seem contradictory—they only seem so—in reality, they are not.

Let us start with number two—mutual cooperation. Nurses want a say in patient care issues, so give it to them. If you have not already done so, establish subcommittees in every department with which nurses interact to obtain goods and services for patients. There should be committees for nursing, pharmacy, dietary, housekeeping, lab, radiology, materiels-management, quality assurance, transport, unit service management, maintenance, ER, OR, ICU, CCU, etc.

Professional nurses need to share in how they are governed, so set up a shared governance committee. Be sure the governor of all committees—the group leader—is an excellent time manager, who starts and ends meetings she chairs on time and keeps the ball rolling. It is a good idea to have a time management consultant in to teach team leaders or meeting chairs how to start and end a meeting on time and to get the most out of participants in the shortest time possible. Otherwise everyone will be "meetinged" to death. The more power you give your staff, the less power they will seek elsewhere, and the more energy they will have to focus on patient-centered care.

EXHIBIT 4.1 | *Clauses of a Sample Nurses Association Contract*

Association Status, Professional Practitioner Status, Employee Status, Work Time, Monetary Benefits—Compensation for time worked and Compensation for Time Not Worked, Unpaid Time Off, Monetary Benefits—Insurance, Monetary Benefits Miscellaneous, Health and Safety, Employee Obligation, Grievance and Arbitration, Business Management, Miscellany, Continuation of Benefits, Effective Date and Duration, Termination, Schedule A Base Rate Compensation Memoranda of Agreements covering various issues including pay checks, staffing, status changes, work schedules, non-nursing functions, shift differentials, premium pay, and the like. Management's Rights.

SUMMARY

This chapter dealt with issues pertinent to labor and management, and especially to labor management cooperation. The overarching theme was that when employees believe they cannot get fair treatment from management, along with lack of job satisfaction, they often seek representation from a third party.

- The Wagner Act of 1935 and the Taft-Hartley Act of 1947 (National Labor Relations Act [NLRA]) established structure for collective bargaining in the United States of America.
- The National Labor Relations Board (NLRB) was established to oversee labor-related issues in the United States of America.
- Union-organizing campaigns: remember TIPS—*Threaten, Interrogate, Promise,* or *Spy*—spells out what the employer may *not* do during a union organizing campaign.
- Mandatory collective bargaining subjects include salary, benefits, and other conditions of employment. The parties must bargain in good faith but are not required to reach agreement.
- Employer may put into effect proposals it made during negotiations if impasse is reached.
- Grievance and discipline—take the high road but maintain a *patient-centered focus.* You do not have to be *mean* to *mean* what you say. Follow the contract and your personnel policies.

▨ Union/management cooperation can even take place where conflict, divergence, and strikes occurred in the recent past—if managers do not take strikes personally.

▨ Before and during labor actions: it is important for management to treat unionized employees as members of the team—even on picket lines— they will return after strikes as members of the team.

▨ Section 2(11) of the National Labor Relations Act (NLRA) defines:

Statutory Supervisory Responsibilities under NLRA: "Having authority, in the interest of the employer, to hire, transfer, suspend, lay off, recall, promote, discharge, assign, reward, or discipline other employees; or responsibly to direct them, or to adjust their grievances, or effectively to recommend such action. If in connection with the foregoing, the exercise of such authority is not of a merely routine or clerical nature, but requires the use of independent judgment."

CHAPTER ENDNOTES

Children's Habilitation Center, Inc., Petitioner, Cross-Respondent, v. National Labor Relations Board, Respondent, Cross-Petitioner. Nos. 88-2538, 88-2735. http://ftp.resource. org/courts.gov/c/F2/887/887.F2d.130.88-2735.88-2538.html. (BNA) 2780, 113 Lab.Cas. P 11,631. Argued September 8, 1989. Decided October 13, 1989.

Forman, H. and G. Davis. 2002. The anatomy of a union campaign. *JONA* 32(9):444–447.

Forman, H. and H. Krauss. 2003. Management's role when employees rethink unionization. *JONA* 33(6):316.

Forman, H. and F. Merrick. 2003. Discipline: Learning the rules of the management high road. *JONA* 33(2):65–67.

Forman, H. and T. Powell. 2003. Union-management cooperation. *JONA* 33(12):621–623.

New Jersey RNs Working Together. http://en.rnsworkingtogether.net/ (accessed July 20, 2010). New Jersey RNs Working Together is a coalition of five unions representing nurses throughout the state. The unions include 1199J, NUHHCE/AFSCME, HPAE/AFT, NJNU/CWA, JNESO/IUOE, and USW.

Peters, T. J. and R. H. Waterman. 2004. *In search of excellence*. New York: Harper Collins.

RNs Working Together. http://www.afscme.org/publications/13205.cfm (accessed July, 20, 2010). RNs Working Together is a coalition of 10 AFL-CIO unions representing more than 200,000 registered nurses and is the largest organization of working nurses in America.

Statutory Supervisory Responsibilities. "Employment Law Alert: Who is a 'Supervisor'?" http://www.stoel.com/index.aspx (accessed May 20, 2010).

Taft-Hartley Labor Act of 1947. http://www.civics-online.org.

United States Court of Appeals, Seventh Circuit. www.ca7.uscourts.gov (accessed March 25, 2010). Argued September 8, 1989. Decided October 13, 1989.

Wagner Act of 1935. http://en.wikipedia.org/wiki/National_Labor_Relations_Act.
Weingarten Rights. "No Right to Representation for Accused Nonunion Employees in Workplace Investigations—But for How Long?" *Workplace Investigation Blog*, http://www.workplaceinvestigationblog.com (accessed February 21, 2010).

5

Personality Traits—The Keys to the Kingdom

If a man does not keep pace with his companions, perhaps it is because he hears a different drummer. Let him step to the music which he hears, however measured or far away. —*Henry David Thoreau*

Vignette I Am Ready, God!

The elderly patient lies quietly in her bed asking God to take her. She is very thin, wraith-like, and barely makes a dent in the mattress. The nurse enters the room and takes her hand. "Frances," she says in a jolly voice, "how are you today?" Frances whispers, "Why doesn't God take me?"

The nurse—an extrovert by nature—says: "Don't talk like that, Frances, God isn't ready to take you." She offers Frances some water. Frances clamps her lips and jaw tightly shut.

The nurse straightens out the bedding while clucking her tongue against her teeth disapprovingly. When she finishes fussing around the room she turns back to Frances and prepares her few medications. Frances turns her face to the wall.

Personality

According to Webster, *Personality* refers to the complex of characteristics that distinguishes an individual . . . *especially* the totality of an individual's behavioral and emotional characteristics *and* that individual's set of distinctive traits and characteristics.

Clearly, in the opening vignette, the nurse assigned to the elderly patient, with a diagnosis of *Failure to Thrive*, did not overcome her upbeat personality to provide care to Frances in a reflective manner. Instead, she imposed her personality, concerns, and objectives onto the patient, thus further burdening a dying woman. In this case, the nurse intervened

143

in order to meet the nurse's needs and not in response to her patient's needs.

Vignette   Invisibility Is Not an Option

It was about an hour into the shift. As usual, the unit—within the postsurgical step down division—was extremely busy, and there had been two call-ins. One had been covered with a per diem, the other remained open.

Suddenly, a supervisor appeared on the unit. Every staff nurse there attempted to become invisible while the supervisor examined the assignment sheet. As she made her way to the nurse manager's area, the entire staff held their breath. Soon, only one nurse seemed to be the focus of attention and she was becoming more and more tense. But that did not last long because the supervisor immediately said to her, "You'll have to float."

There was no discussion; no call for volunteers; no chance for the nurse to object or explain why she should not be chosen to float; nothing other than an order, and it was delivered by the supervisor instead of by the unit nurse manager.

Protocol was breached, the nurse manager's authority was undermined, and authoritarianism ruled the day.

Combine Art and Science—Predict Success

It did not have to be this way. Selecting appropriate staff to float to understaffed units, especially after they have already started their shift elsewhere, or to serve effectively on teams is both an art and a science. It requires recognition and classification of technical skills and of personality traits that will predict success. Identifying technical skills is the easy part and is built into most health care organizations' orientation and continuing education programs. Ascertaining personality traits as they pertain to specific assignments and to team cooperation is another matter.

Creative teams are needed everywhere in the health delivery environment. The Joint Commission requires evidence of team effectiveness. One of the core values of magnet qualification is teamwork. The challenge is not in the *doing* as much as in the *preparing* to do.

Every day, leaders work with many types of individuals. The idea is to fit round pegs into round holes. There are those individuals who respond well to a highly structured environment and some who want to wing it; there are the go getters and the procrastinators; the action oriented and those who analyze and evaluate before they get started. There are the companionable individuals and the loners, the creators and the copiers. Some have insight and intuition, and others are hardworking and task oriented. If you pick the loner, for example, and assign her to greet new graduates, you have set up a probable failure, or, if too many of one type and none or too few of another are selected for a team, these simple stylistic differences can cause coworkers to lock horns and bring projects to a grinding halt. Paradoxically, these same differences in how individuals communicate, make decisions, address conflict, and solve problems, when properly combined and channeled, are the building blocks of the most well-rounded and effective teams. The question is: How does one effectively type personalities within the health care employment setting—when there is little time, and some people do not readily reveal their basic personae?

Vignette   The Tortoise and the Hare

This is a well-known story that can easily be applied to just about any health care setting. It is about a race between two creatures—one known to sprint, and the other to creep along. They are contestants in a lengthy race. Most bettors put their money on the sprinter—the hare—but he falters from fatigue because he does not conserve his energy for the long haul. The tortoise, on the other hand, ambles along and gets the job done—slowly but surely.

I am not suggesting that we employ a bunch of amblers in our fast-paced health care environments. However, there is a place for people of all manners and styles—assuming they are identified and situated in jobs that suit their personalities. Some folks reveal themselves readily. They speak and move slowly and maybe even think slowly. I would not assign them to the fast-paced emergency services, but I might place them in hospice, dialysis, or geriatrics.

Sprinters reveal themselves pretty readily as well. But what about the rest? Dr. Carl Gustav Jung's work on the psychology of personality types has been used extensively as a team-building tool. Isabel Briggs Myers and her mother Katharine Briggs—together known as Myers/Briggs (MB)—found Jung's work useful in developing a method to measure personality types as they apply to forming effective work groups. They believed that seemingly random variations in the behavior of individuals are really methodical and consistent because of basic differences in the way individuals distinguish one thing from another—in the way they perceive and are perceived.

Remember, perception—or the way you feel about someone or something—is a funny thing in that it is so personal. That is why we keep coming back to it. Just look around and see some people wearing sweaters and other people sweating. Note that the temperature in the area is the same—but individuals *perceive* it and *react* to it differently.

We keep asking questions like, how does it *feel* to be a patient on your unit? Or, how does it *feel* to be a staff member under your leadership? In team building, Myers/Briggs used perception combined with judgment as part of their model to help build effective teams. They believed that human behavior is predictable, and they based this on *Type theory*, which hearkens back to Jung. Type theory proposes that human behavior may be classified and made accessible for study and application to practice. So they developed the Myers–Briggs Type Indicator Instrument (MBTII). According to this theory, everyone is born predisposed to certain personality types. Some people are Extraverted and typed by MB as (E). If they are Introverted, they are labeled (I). If they are predominantly Sensing, they get an (S), and if they rely mostly on intuition, they are an (N). So that person is known as an E-I-S-N.

These characteristics are then added to the qualities of Thinking (T) or Feeling (F), and Judging (J) or Perceiving (P). So ultimately, an individual may be classified as ESFJ—someone who is (E) extraverted; (S) senses rather than intuits; problem solves by (F) feeling rather than thinking; and (J) judges rather than perceives. No values are placed on these qualities; none are better than the others. They all just *are*, and importantly, a good mix within a work group ensures a well-rounded team.

In a related approach, Dr. Max Wideman, of the Stevens Institute of Technology in New Jersey (Wideman, 2006), is on the same page with Meyers/Briggs. But he takes it a step further. He suggests that certain personality types are suited to specific jobs—if *appropriately assigned*. If improperly assigned, however, they become negative influences. To illustrate his point, he employs terms such as: Explorer, Coordinator, Driver, and Administrator. As you might imagine, the explorer is a visionary who is future oriented, while the coordinator is mission oriented and a conflict mediator.

According to Wideman, the driver and administrator, when properly assigned, could not be better at their jobs. But when placed in the wrong assignments, they can cause much trouble. Let us take the administrator, for example. An individual with this personality type tends to be objective and analytic. While focused on solutions, the administrator is a decision maker who readily implements those decisions.

Does this not sound like the right person for a management track? But if you assign this person to a subordinate position—one in which she has to follow someone less astute than she, less goal directed and slow to implement decisions, then this individual just might seem overzealous, stubborn, judgmental, and hypercritical.

When surfing the Internet by Googling *team building* and *personality typing*, I found pages and pages of information about the subjects. Most of what I found, both MB and other similar methods, was Jungian based. The often misunderstood terms extrovert and introvert derive from his work. In Jung's original usage, the extravert—not necessarily the loud, party girl, is someone who finds meaning outside the self, in the surrounding world. The introvert, on the other hand, is meditative and seeks meaning from within.

This is important for the patient-centered manager to know when making assignments. Would a meditative introvert not be a good choice to bring an atmosphere of peace and understanding to a dying patient? How about choosing an extravert to consider a float assignment or greeting new employees?

The authors, Joanne Walter and Ardeshir Bayat, known for their work in personality typing and neurolinguistic programming write that "knowing what personality type you are [or are members of your staff] can benefit you and your appreciation of others." They have a method similar to MB, and as well, they seek to reveal the extrovert/introvert, sensation, intuition, thinking, feeling, judging, and perceiving, aspects of the individuals being tested. Like many personality tests, it is Jungian based.

If you want to take an online test, there is a website for your convenience (Personality Test Center, 2009). It is similar to Myers–Briggs though less complex. You might find it useful and you might find it fun.

If you decide to learn something about the personality types of your team, think about a couple of things before you get started. Discuss this idea with them and engage their cooperation. Invite their input, and, as I mentioned before, make it enjoyable. If you have a psychiatric department—staff psychiatrist, psychologist, or psychiatric nurse practitioner or social worker—with whom to collaborate, by all means, take advantage of their specialized knowledge. Perhaps one of them knows of a personality typing method you could investigate together.

Once you have this information—use it. Use it for team building. Use it for planning assignments. Remember the old adage: If you do not use it, you lose it, and then you have wasted an important resource.

THE TIP OF THE ICEBERG

Another significant field of behavioral study from which to seek an understanding of human behavior is that of Sigmund Freud, who preceded Jung. Understanding Freud's *topography of the mind* using an iceberg as a visual illustration, might help the manager better grasp the meaning of a staff member's unexpected emotional outburst to certain issues and stressors. According to Freud, there are three levels of consciousness:

- The conscious, which corresponds to the tip of the iceberg—10%. This is the part of the mind that contains our awareness. We can verbalize our conscious experiences and think about them in logical fashion.
- The preconscious, 10–15%, which corresponds to the middle of the iceberg. It is larger than the tip, but not as large as the base. This is ordinary memory, which can readily be brought into consciousness.
- The unconscious, 75–80%, which corresponds to the base of the iceberg. This is the enormous underwater portion that, in real life, is the bane of sailors. Freud believed this is inaccessible to conscious awareness. He thought of it as a dumping ground for urges, feelings, and ideas tied to anxiety, conflict, and pain. Further, he believed that these unconscious urges, feelings, and ideas exerted influence on our actions and conscious awareness and that this is where the work of the Id, Ego, and Superego takes place. Freud posited that material passes easily back and forth between the conscious and the preconscious and can slip into the unconscious. Truly unconscious material, according to Freud, is inaccessible to the individual without the guidance of a psychoanalyst.

Vignette "That's My Face!?!"

The CNE of a large unionized skilled nursing facility received repeated complaints about a CNA whose facial expression was described in terms including mean, stern, angry, frightening, hostile, intimidating, aggressive, and belligerent. She had worked for the organization for about 5 years, and there were no complaints about her work, attendance, or anything other than her facial expression and demeanor. She had been repeatedly counseled but denied understanding what anyone was referring to. She kept saying, "That's my face."

Patients feared her and did not want her to care for them. Family members and social service staff alike had been to nursing administration and to the CEO demanding that her employment be terminated.

The CNE made an appointment to see her. She positioned herself behind her desk as the aide entered the office and took a seat folding her arms across her ample bosom. She had a scowl on her face and indeed looked quite frightening. Her brow was knitted; her eyes squinted; her mouth pursed; the sides of her jaw tight with her cheek muscles knotted into prominent bulges. Even her nostrils flared.

Without a word, the CNE reached under her desk and withdrew a 20-inch round mirror and placed it in front of the aide and asked, "If you were ill, debilitated, and dependent, would you like to be greeted and cared for by that person?"

The nurse aide burst into tears.

Removing the mirror and pushing a box of tissues across the desk, the CNE waited. Finally, the aide calmed down and looked at her director who remained silent.

The CNA said, "My God, I had no idea I looked like that. How could that be me? No wonder no one wanted me to care for them. I'm so ashamed. . . ." and she started to cry again.

This time, the CNE arose from her chair and walked around her desk to the NA's side. She placed her hand upon the woman's shoulder in a comforting manner as she thought about the problem. It seems there was a long history to this situation—one that went back long before the CNE arrived at the facility. The more the nurse aide was counseled, the more upset she became. The more upset she became, the angrier she got. The angrier she got, the more she showed it on her face and in her posture, and so, a vicious cycle was born—until the CNE decided a picture was worth a thousand words.

With her agreement, this aide was transferred to a nonpatient care assignment in which she did not have to face patients who already had decided they did not want to interact with her. Management staff was counseled about the value of treating this employee with kindness, which, over time, started her on the road to recovery.

Although she did not return to patient care, she relaxed and seemed to enjoy her new work assignment. In a while, the stress and worry lines in her face eased and so did her tense expression and bearing. As these things happened, people stopped avoiding her and she developed trust.

In this case, the simple act of placing a mirror in front of a stressed, defensive employee instead of bombarding her with harsh words literally changed her life—from that of a lonely, angry unhappy human being to one who was readmitted to a social circle of her peers. Empathy and out-of-the-box thinking went a long way.

We do not really know the etiology of the nurse aide's visage and behavior. But if we refer to Freud's concepts, we must look at things like ego strength and early childhood. These are factors that affect us all. They help mold our personalities and make us what we become as adults.

TYPING PERSONALITIES WITH A CLICK OF A MOUSE

You do not have to be Myers–Briggs experts or use Wideman's descriptives to type your staff members' personalities or go through expensive complex rigamaroles to figure out your own. You can turn to the Internet to find resources to test yourself—*if* you do not already know yourself. Try the Web site I mentioned earlier or seek another (Neurolinguistic Programming, 2009) if you want to find out who you are—or more likely to validate what you already know. If you want to have a little fun—download a free Jungian-based personality test from the Internet, and set up a conference with your staff. Make it voluntary and make it fun. After some discussion, ask staff members to make a note of their personality types and then have volunteers take and grade their own tests. Most people are right on the mark—or close to it.

When I have done this as a consultant, the room rang with laughter. Nurses are often found to be high in the "feeling" and "intuition" range, so be prepared to nurture those "analytical" types when you find them. This is because when building an effective team, too many of one type and not enough of another will not only result in an unbalanced team, it will also result in skewed outcomes. But sometimes you are in for a surprise.

Vignette   **The Taurus and the Sag—Or the Rat and the Dragon**

Do you believe in astrology? According to my friend Webster, "Astrology is the divination of the supposed influences of the stars and planets on human affairs and terrestrial events by their positions and aspects. And Astrologers are those who practice Astrology."

Astrologers with intricate knowledge of the heavens, and the juxtaposition of the moon, the sun, the planets, and other related things, make certain predictions about you, your relationships, and your future. Investigate this field and you will learn of 12 signs of the Zodiac that match the constellations as they existed around 2000 years ago (see chapter endnotes for Zodiac URL).

Each sign has appended to it the energy qualities of earth, fire, air, or water. There also are *personality traits* that attach to each of these signs of the Zodiac. As a result, certain personality matchups would be predicted to be favorable—or unfavorable—between and among people born under those signs.

Here is a personal example: In Western astrology, Taurus—a fixed sign (my husband)—and Sagittarius—a mutable sign (that's me)—are *not* predicted to make the greatest match for matrimony. But in Chinese astrology, we are a Dragon and a Rat (clever creature), and we are predicted to be the perfect couple—and here we are more than 33 years later and still going strong. I wonder what our matchup would be anticipated to be in Vedic astrology.

I'm not suggesting we consult an astrologer and cast everyone's chart, but I am advocating for managers to recognize the importance of matching personality to assignment whenever possible. Think about how you might employ personality typing—or at least consider personalities of the team members in your organization when you plan new units or devise team composition, make float assignments, and review change of assignment requests. When you see people at odds with one another, maybe a personality type review might help you help them resolve their issues. Personality clashes do not make for productive encounters.

In any event, brush up on Jungian psychology and add a little Freud to the mix. Then broaden your scope by also moving into the realms of study of the many critics of Freud and Jung. Among them were *Humanistic* personality theorists (and later behavioral aficionados). They objected to the determinism of Freudian models. Determinism posits that things are *determined* or *caused* by that which came before. There are even those who believe that past life experiences influence behavior in the present existence. For more information, use Google as your search engine or any one that you favor. The name Brian Weiss might focus your search.

SWITCH GEARS FOR A MORE MODERN APPROACH

As we moved deeper into the twentieth century, personal experience, or *phenomenology*, and *self-actualization* or the fulfillment of human potential seemed more important than concern with psychosexual development and the subconscious—Freud's areas of inquiry. These all are interesting fields of study for nurse leaders. We are in the business of motivating people and encouraging them to heights of expanding achievement. Understanding what makes people tick from the many perspectives of the various schools of psychology can only help to reinforce our knowledge base. The vast reach of the Internet brings enormous amounts of information into our homes at the touch of a mouse. Once you open the doors to the mind, however, be prepared to spend time there. It is a fascinating place to browse, and it can help you be more effective at one of your most important responsibilities—ensuring the correct placement of staff members and well-balanced teams.

What could be better than that? Perhaps nothing, but here is something that could be just as good.

Vignette   At Ease, Please

The director is late for an interview through no fault of her own. A major accident on a bridge had stopped traffic dead in its tracks. Her car is stuck in the midst of the worst traffic jam ever. She uses her cell phone to call ahead. The secretary says she has a 2-hour window of opportunity. By the time she arrives at her destination, there are only 15 minutes left for her to interview for the most important position of her career. "What to do, what to do?" She keeps repeating to herself as she parks her car, freshens her lipstick, and races to the building.

Believing that the interviewer would have read her cover letter and resumé, she quickly decides to employ neurolinguistic mirroring—a technique she had recently learned about. Believing it will maximize her chances of landing this very important position that she believes she can ace, she hones her five senses in preparation to be ushered in to the inner sanctum—the office of the director.

As she enters the room, she quickly takes in everything she sees—color of walls, drapes, furnishings, position of desk and chair, flowers, plants, photos, certificates and degrees, and especially where they are positioned in regard to the desk and the door. She also assesses paintings, odors, sounds, and the type of fabrics favored by the occupant. In a quick world of instant assessment—everything matters.

Then she notes how she is greeted and whether or not the director retreats behind her desk or sits next to her. She works at evaluating what kind of individual this person is—introverted or extraverted; formal or informal; family oriented or business oriented—or both.

As she absorbs this, she seats herself in the chair as indicated and assumes a formal upright position with both feet flat on the floor because she interprets the office and its occupant to be formal and business like. She then responds as prompted using the information she has gathered to temper her speech and tone in an effort to place the interviewer at ease and create a receptive environment for herself.

Her responses are truthful, her own questions are to the point, and the interview—albeit abbreviated—goes well and ends on time. She is invited back for a second and more extensive interview. Ultimately, she gets the job.

NEUROLINGUISTICS

Neurolinguistic programming (NLP), according to the Oxford English Dictionary, is "a model of interpersonal communication chiefly concerned with the relationship between successful patterns of behavior and the subjective experiences (especially patterns of thought) underlying them." It first was developed by founders Richard Bandler and John Grinder in the 1970s as a rapid-fire form of psychological therapy for a full range of problems. It was also thought to be an effective method for the development of self-determination through overcoming those limitations one learned through life experiences. Further, it emphasized "well-being" and "healthy functioning."

But NLP has not caught on as a widely used methodology for the treatment of the psychologically impaired because it has not been rigorously tested according to scientific method. It has, however, been offered as a way to increase sales effectiveness. There is an interesting book available through Amazon entitled *The Unfair Advantage* that discusses NLP in this regard. Some people believe NLP to be overly manipulative and therefore unethical.

Here is some information about NLP from *The Unfair Advantage*—you decide.

Fundamentally, NLP skills help you make someone feel comfortable and trust you by using certain techniques that may include mirroring their posture and verbal speed, and recognizing their biases and language preferences. The goal is to establish rapport. In sales, its preliminary goal is to make the sale. In nursing, it is an essential component of trust. In management and leadership, rapport is crucial to any number of things—including establishing trust, building effective teams, leading and motivating individuals and groups, directing and controlling a workforce, building relationships. Rapport is an essential part of building any type of effective workforce.

My question is, even if you mirror certain actions and behaviors of others in an effort to place someone at ease, and your motives are just, is it immoral or unethical? Let us take the vignette that opened this chapter, but this time apply a mirroring technique and see what happens.

Vignette   Am I A Mirror of Your Soul?

The nurse enters the room of a dying patient and says: "How are you today, Mrs. Jones?"

"I'm dying," the patient responds, "how should I feel?"

The nurse, experienced in NLP, says: "You feel like you're dying, Mrs. Jones?"

"I just told you that. Go away," says the patient moaning as she struggles to turn away from the nurse.

"Are you in pain, Mrs. Jones?" asks the nurse, as she gently eases the patient onto her side and smoothes the bed linen. She rests her hand soothingly on Mrs. Jones' shoulder, maintaining human contact.

"Everything hurts," says the patient. "Everything!"

"I'll get you something for pain. You'll soon feel better," says the nurse reassuringly as she quietly withdraws her hand from her patient.

Mrs. Jones sighs as she relaxes—just a little.

Not everyone is able to handle death and dying. It is a specialty unto itself. No seasoned manager would assign a nurse to an ICU patient without vetting the nurse's ability in that area of expertise—so why would anyone do less for a nurse sent to care for a dying patient? The nurse in the above scenario was skillful and sensitive. She knew her field—what to do and what to not do.

As we move on to neurolinguistic programming, we have a method similar to the reflective techniques the nurse used to mirror what was in Mrs. Jones' heart, mind, and soul as she struggled with what little life she had remaining to her so close to her death.

The nurse reflected Mrs. Jones' feelings back to her and said, "You feel as if you're dying?" This validated Mrs. Jones' feelings. Then, in response to her moans, she offered medication and comfort.

In sales calls, interactions, or interviews as in the opening vignette, the person skilled in this technique scans the environment of the client or the room of a patient and notices small things about him. Is he formal or informal? Does he sit behind his desk or next to his callers? Is his jacket on or off? What are his handshake and speech patterns like? The nurse manager or client then uses this information to set the patient, or staff member, or whomever, at ease and to enhance communication.

For those readers who are wondering why I am covering sales calls—nurse managers are always selling. We sell—or convince, teach, promote, market, and persuade—others in their pursuit of excellence. So let us go back to techniques of mirroring or as the psychologist Carl Rogers called it, *reflective interviewing*. This is a therapeutic way to learn what the interviewee has on his mind by restating what the person has said—as in the above example—instead of occupying the airwaves with the interviewer's thoughts. As you can imagine, persons with certain personality types might do this more easily than others.

SUMMARY

This chapter defines personality as a complex of characteristics that distinguishes an individual. This simple definition leads the reader to a series of stories, thoughts, actions, and inactions that impact either positively or negatively on patient-centered care.

- Considering personality traits when selecting individuals for assignments such as floating. For example, those individuals who like to travel—the adventurer—may do better floating than do homebodies.
- Selecting a good mix of various personality types when building effective teams helps ensure success.
- Methods of typing personality are reviewed, with Carl Gustave Jung's work as a basis for understanding.
- Myers–Briggs—MBTI for Myers–Briggs Type Indicator—is a well-known personality typing method based on Jung's work. Katharine Cook Briggs and her daughter, Isabel Briggs Myers, produced an instrument to measure personality type.
- Myers and Briggs believed that everyone is born predisposed to personality preferences: extraverted, introverted, sensing, intuiting . . .
- Although Sigmund Freud preceded Jung, in this chapter, he follows. Freud is well-known (among other things) for his study of the unconscious mind and its effect on behavior.
- Among other things, Freud posited that behavior may be influenced by things stored in the unconscious portion of the human mind.
- The more the existential manager knows about this field of study, the less off balance she will be when, seemingly out of the blue, a staff member appears to overreact to a situation.
- Personality, facial expression, and neurolinguistic programming make up a threesome in this chapter.
- Neurolinguistic programming is presented as a method to be used to place others at ease in patient care, at interviews, and for many other interpersonal situations.
- Psychologist Carl Rogers wrote extensively about reflective interviewing as a technique to enhance communication in revealing the thoughts, feelings, and actions of others to help relieve burdens and fears—of pain and suffering, of dying, of decision making.

CHAPTER ENDNOTES

Freud, S. *Topography of the mind*. http://wilderdom.com/personality/L8-3Topography MindIceberg.html (accessed December 19, 2009).

Jung Typology Test. http//www.humanmetrics.com/cgi-win/JTypes2.asp (accessed January 30, 2010).

Meyers Briggs. *Type Indicator Instrument*. http://www.infotech.com/ITA/Research% 20Centers/Project20%/Project20%Teams/A%20Great%20Tool%20for%20Building %20Teams%20-%20Personality%20Typing.aspx (accessed May 2, 2006).

Neurolinguistic Programming. http://archive.student.bmj.com/issues/03/06/life/206.php (accessed December 9, 2009).

Personality Test Center. http://www.personalitytest.net/types/index.htm (accessed December 9, 2009).

Wideman, M. http//www.maxwideman.com/papers/success/together.htm (accessed May 15, 2006).

Zodiac. http://www.referencecenter.com/ref/dictionary?invocationType=topsearchbox. refcentre&query=zodiac (accessed March 25, 2010).

6

Bridging the Cultural Divide

We are each of us angels with only one wing, and we can only fly by embracing one another. —*Luciano de Crescenzo*

Vignette   God Is Everywhere

My Jewish father lay dying in a Catholic Hospice. He had been moved there from the hospital's coronary care unit when all that could be done for him had been done.

Dad had been born into Jewish orthodoxy, had lived his life as a conservative Jew, adhering to its tenets and giving charitably to those who needed it.

Now at nearly 97 years of age—or 96 point 10 as he liked to say—he was spending his final hours in the Catholic facility under the personal care of his Southern Baptist private aides, open bibles in hand. Their favorite televangelist was preaching from the TV mounted on the wall above a gleaming Crucifix.

Our loving hands rested on my father as he peacefully drew his last breath. No one moved, and time was suspended until I set it in motion by leaning over and kissing my father farewell, wishing him a safe journey. I embraced each aide and thanked them one by one. They closed their bibles and departed.

Soon a nun entered the room. She held me for a moment and asked if she could say a prayer.

"Old Testament, please, Sister," I responded.

She murmured the 23rd Psalm—"The Lord is my shepherd. I shall not want . . ."

The silence in the room deepened as she concluded: "Amen."

Turning quietly away, she exited leaving me alone with the man I had known and loved throughout my life and who now was gone.

As I waited alone with my father I wondered, "Where were the nurses?"

I telephoned my sister in New York. We cried together for a while. We would see each other before long in New York for dad's funeral.

In a few moments, a priest arrived. We had become friends during my father's hospitalization. We chatted and then he left me alone to wait and wonder. Where was everyone? I thought I might have entered the Twilight Zone, so to pass the time, I started a crossword puzzle in the *New York Times* that my husband had left in the room. He had taken my stepmother to her home to prepare for the trip north.

Soon, a Rabbi arrived. I started to think about who might have notified him but was interrupted by his asking me if he could "cover" my father.

Momentarily confused I said "he is covered" referring to the sheet and blanket snugly tucked in around Dad.

"No," he said "In our religion we cover the face of the dead."

"Right," I thought, "I knew that." I just did not have the heart to cover my father's face. "Of course, Rabbi, please do." I said as I positioned myself at my father's head while the Rabbi performed this rite. He then asked if he could say a prayer, and with my permission, he did.

Dad would say he had a terrific send-off: Baptist, Pentecostal if you count the Televangelist, Catholic, and finally, Jewish. He had a great sense of humor and fine intercultural acceptance and understanding, which he passed on to my sister and to me.

Finally, representatives of the funeral home arrived and took my father away. I followed them to the door of the hospital, and there, I had no choice but to let him go. Not once did I see a nurse during this time of his dying and his death, and I still wonder why.

Here is another intercultural story—this time in a skilled nursing facility (SNF). In this scenario, hard feelings were generated due to lack of knowledge about the origin of a custom. This ignorance caused deep affront to some nurse aides. As often happens, insult turns into anger and anger into seething resentment. See what you think about it and what you might have done—first to have prevented it and second to fix what had become broken.

Vignette   Had They Only Known . . .

A group of nurse aides—African American Christians—were extremely upset. They had been caring for an orthodox Jewish patient for several years. As was common practice, each had assumed responsibility for total care of the patient or resident, as was the common nomenclature for occupants of the facility. This included bathing, toileting, feeding, dressing, ambulating, and similar services.

They had a good relationship both with the patient and with his family members and suffered a loss upon his death. Without explanation, they were told by their supervisor that they were not to provide post mortem care—readying his body to be removed by the funeral home attendants.

At first the aides were hurt. Then they became angry. They articulated their feelings to each other this way: "What's the matter? We were good enough to clean him up when he was alive. Why are we not good enough now that he's dead?"

Had there been a program in the facility addressing intercultural understanding, the aides would have been assured that indeed they were good enough. It really had nothing to do with that. Instead, because of the long history of desecration of Jewish corpses going back through the ages, orthodox Jews and others had as their custom that only other Jews could provide such services. It had become a cultural norm.

CULTURAL NORMS AND OTHER THINGS . . .

In some cultures, the eldest male is the leader of the family, so it is important to address him with questions and instructions about health information. In some cultures, the eldest female is the matriarch.

Some cultures prize modesty and some could not care less. There are those whose smile is their umbrella and those who connect other facial expressions with warmth or similar positive emotions.

Tone of voice, body language, gender, sex, sexual orientation, age, body type, social space, eye contact, touch, social class, disability, hair type and color, eye shape and shade—the list is seemingly endless. All of it, and more, matter. Are you a member of the working class or upper class? Are you a doctor or a nurse? A professor or a student?

Vignette   We Are Doctors, Too

Five women were waiting for the maître d' to escort them to their table in a four-star restaurant. They had made reservations and were on time. All were professors in a nearby Ivy League university. Suddenly, four men entered the restaurant and diverted the attention of the maître d'. One of the women stepped up and said, "Excuse me."

Officiously, the maître d' replied, "But Madame, these gentlemen are busy doctors."

The woman replied, "Allow me to introduce you to my companions—all busy doctors, too: Doctor Smith, Doctor Jones, Doctor Harris, Doctor Able, and I am Doctor Evans. Since we were here first, kindly seat us first."

I and many of my female, doctorally prepared colleagues have found that when we introduce ourselves as "Doctor," we are asked what our medical specialty is. If we say nursing or nursing administration or education, the person rapidly reverts to using "Ms.," especially in a physician's office. The one place this does not seem to happen is in academe where the culture recognizes nonmedical doctorates. Society has a long way to go.

Here is another story to help drive home that point.

Vignette   Do Not Call Me Boy!

We were a small nursing administrative staff working out of miniscule office in a long-term care facility that was slated to close. It was the sponsoring agency for a brand new, modern, building that was being prepared to receive the 100 or so patients who had called this place home for many years. They would soon be joined by more than 400 patients to be admitted over the coming months once the new building was completed and all services were up and running.

The old facility had fallen into disrepair and was decrepit and uninviting. There was an entirely new nurse administrative staff—four of us consisting of the CNE, an ADN for Education, a nurse manager, and me. I was in charge of nursing services in the old facility.

The original plan was that we would only be in this building for 3 months. But in reality, 3 months began to stretch into what would likely be at least 6 or 7 months. So we agreed we needed to spruce up the place with a fresh coat of paint to make it more attractive to potential employees.

After much ado, we prevailed upon the boss to approve not only the job but the overtime necessary to have it accomplished over the weekend. However, on Saturday afternoon, a "weekend" administrator called and rescinded the approval—while the painters were working. Both painters were furious.

When we arrived Monday morning, we found the men working at a snail's pace. Their anger was palpable. No one could blame them for their fury. Being called at 11 A.M. Saturday morning to be told to clock out after having received approval to work was totally unacceptable.

Everyone sympathized with them, but there was only one nursing office. In her effort to speed them along, the nurse manager—well-meaning, white, and unprejudiced—entered the office and said to the two African American painters, "Gee, boys, you're doing such a great job." A look of sheer wrath come over the face of one of the painters as he turned toward her and literally leaped off his ladder, lunging at her. In his mind—based on an imperception brought on by decades of racism—she had called him "boy."

The CNE stepped between them and put up her hands shouting "Stop! She did not mean any disrespect! Please, allow her to explain. Please!"

Discussion

During and after the gruesome days when men and women were kept in slavery and well into the twentieth century, especially in the South, the word "boy" was used to address adult black men. It is not only a racial slur but a term replete with the degradation that accompanies being owned by another. This painter had already been insulted by first having been told it was all right to put in overtime, then having that permission withdrawn in the middle of the weekend—by a white man. Now, he thought he heard a white woman call him "boy." His breaking point had been reached.

Remember the story I told in the section on inference/observation confusion about a white patient who escaped from a locked psychiatric unit? That man managed to exit the hospital and sprint into an all-white neighborhood.

Two black orderlies gave chase—wearing street clothes.

The good folks in their houses looked out their windows and saw these two black men chasing a white man and . . . remember? They called the police. The police answered the call to duty and came and arrested the two orderlies. In the meantime, the escaped patient got away. In this case, the orderlies took no offense. But I would not have blamed them if they had. Would you?

RELIGION AS A DRIVING FORCE

Religion has been a strong motivator for action throughout man's history. It has been a cause of many charitable acts—feeding the hungry, clothing the poor, educating and bringing health care to the needy, and so on. Unfortunately, it also has caused destruction and mayhem through war, migration, mass killings, and attempts at genocide. Religion has touched every facet of human history and life. Man falls to his knees in awe, withstands torture, forfeits his life, or rises to heights of charitable giving.

Each day brings new things, and in the areas of little known cultures and religious practices, new things can be very interesting indeed.

Vignette   Special Delivery

The wife of a Gypsy king was in labor. The entire tribe of 23 people had camped out in the hospital lobby. Security called the patient care administrator and anxiously reported that they were attempting to light a bonfire in some wastebaskets they had gathered for that purpose. Upon investigating, it was learned that a bonfire was an important part of the "birthing ritual" without which the Gypsies were certain the child would be stillborn. They were as frantic as were hospital security personnel.

Remembering that the adjacent Skilled Nursing Facility (SNF) had a barbecue pit on its back patio, the administrator assured the Gypsy king that arrangements could be made.

They were soon escorted to the SNF's patio where they were assisted in securing what they needed to complete their ritual. Shortly thereafter, a healthy baby boy was born to the Gypsy queen and everyone was thrilled. Patient-centered care was accomplished and, obviously, the ritual was effective.

Discussion

When it comes to culture and religion, there are no rights, there are no wrongs; there are only misunderstandings bred from ignorance and prejudice. The very word prejudice defines itself—to "pre" judge—often without rhyme or reason. For example, New Yorkers are often prejudged to be unfriendly and rude, and yet when the Twin Towers came down, they rushed by the scores to help total strangers, putting their own lives on the line, and many were injured or killed.

African Americans were prejudged to be ignorant and lazy and therefore unable to properly care for their families without welfare or make the climb out of the ghettos. But now we have a black president, and black physicians, lawyers, professors, astronauts, Supreme Court judges, and other "ordinary" citizens who are successful and contributive members of society.

Gays are thought by some people to be unable to serve in the military without causing major disruptions, and yet, in Western Europe, Israel, and also in the American Armed Forces, albeit surreptitiously, gays and others who are not a part of the heterosexual majority serve meritoriously.

Jews are thought to be penurious; Irish drunkards; Italians gangsters. Does that apply to *all* of the individuals who fall within those categories? The problem is that many people who think these things may believe just that. If they do, they may treat all people within the group as though they fit these definitions. Then, they themselves are thought of and treated as rednecks, or worse.

The week before I wrote these words, a white supremacist walked into the Holocaust Museum in our nation's capital and shot dead an African American security guard. The shooter had already served time in prison for other acts of violence and was well known for his vicious, prejudicial views. But the law protected him and exposed others to deadly harm.

We hear of kids going on the rampage and assaulting people they hate over differences in race, color, religion, sexual orientation, and other issues. Presumably, they were taught these attitudes in their homes, schools, and playgrounds. These attitudes are reflected in the care, or lack of care, delivered in our health care facilities. It is also present in the relationships between nursing teams and interdisciplinary teams, and no matter what the law states about our obligation to provide culturally competent care, these prejudices interfere day-to-day and minute-to-minute with the delivery of quality services. We of good faith ask: What should patient-centered nurse leaders/managers do?

What follows is a story of conflict within a large institution due to cultural differences but particularly within a nurse management team. The casual bystander would be unlikely to notice any disparity in appearance—these individuals seemed to be similar from a racial perspective. They all spoke English with a lilt—although to the careful listener, there were some differences in cadence and inflection. Their food choices seemed comparable. Yet there were cliques and a palpable lack of cooperation between and among members of these social groupings. Upon consideration, the facts revealed themselves.

Vignette   A Laboratory for Cultural Dissonance

The majority of nursing staff were British West Indian—from Jamaica, Barbados, Trinidad, or Antigua. The rest consisted of about 6% Southern African American, 3% Filipino, 1% White Anglo Saxon Protestant and Catholic, and 1% other. The medical mix was predominantly white Jewish and Christian, Indian, Asian, and other. The patients in the hospital reflected the community: West Indian, African American, and Orthodox and Hassidic Jewish. The nursing home was predominantly Jewish. It was a veritable laboratory for cultural dissonance and for study.

There were numerous problems. Cultural dissonance among and between all levels of staff was manifested, for example, by preferential scheduling. Supervisors were favoring countrymen with prime holiday leave, overtime, and vacation time. This was easy to validate just by looking back at the records. Once he was convinced, the newly appointed CNE was committed to change. He believed that the culture of favoritism had to end. The question was, how would he accomplish it?

He determined that the best people to answer the question were the involved participants, so he opened the issue at a staff meeting. After much debate, a day was set aside for focus groups comprising members of the management team. They were to hash out the problem and produce programs and plans of correction.

The group chose the associate director of education to be their mediator and resource person because she was considered impartial. She was, however, very outspoken. She had not been involved in any disciplinary action. She was middle-aged, Catholic, white, and a first generation American of Italian ancestry. Therefore, she was not of the majority.

Conversation flowed freely despite rivalry between and among people from the different cultures. When contention reared its head and could not be resolved, the ADN interceded.

Ultimately, the group agreed that monthly cultural educational programs would be conducted, during which representatives from a selected culture would prepare foods, costumes, musical demonstrations, posters, and other things to showcase their heritage. Cultures would be rotated on a monthly basis.

This program was well advertised throughout the organization and well attended. In tandem, scheduling of work days and holidays was transferred from unit-based, hand-prepared to a centralized computer system implemented over time. This alone was expected to eliminate most of the favoritism exercised by supervisory personnel.

Educational programs on intercultural understanding, the importance of fairness, overcoming role conflict, and maintaining a patient-centered focus were established as ongoing institutional norms.

These interventions constituted the easy parts of the transition programs. The difficult part was whittling away at deep-seated prejudice, and in many cases, out and out virulent hatred. The CNE accepted that overcoming extreme dislike was unlikely, at least over the short term, so he set his sights on behavioral changes.

Areas of importance that he could objectively quantify included schedules, eye contact, and validated performance appraisals. MBWA led to direct observation, impromptu patient interviews and discussions with nursing staff, physicians, department heads, administrators, and others.

Even those individuals who feign proper behavior cannot sustain it over time unless they have made authentic, lasting change. To do this, they require ongoing reinforcement and positive feedback. Prejudice takes a long time to develop and a longer time to tear down.

Here is another story about deep-seated prejudice against the culture of HIV-AIDS in the gay community. Before caregivers can properly interact with and treat such patients, they first must access and acknowledge such feelings. It is up to the patient-centered nurse managers to help them do so. The methods used can be transposed to any caregiving setting.

Vignette I Am Not Intolerant

She was a consultant about to conduct an all-day seminar with a home care agency regarding HIV/AIDS prejudice among its staff. These were predominantly white, Anglo-Saxon Protestant female RNs and home health aides. Their patients were primarily white and black gay men who were HIV positive or who had full blown AIDS.

After introductions, the consultant asked everyone to close their eyes. Then she asked those who were without prejudice to raise a hand. About 40% of the attendees put a hand in the air.

The consultant then offered a series of scenarios and asked the same question. Sample questions included:

- Your 15-year-old daughter announces she is gay—and pregnant. Are you upset?
- Your white son announces he is engaged to a black girl, or a black man.
- Your daughter announces she is transgender and plans gender reassignment.

Many more questions were asked along these lines until the naysayers admitted to an area or two of narrow-mindedness. After each example, the percentage of admittedly prejudiced participants rose until finally, only one person out of the nearly 75 could not be pushed over the prejudice line.

At this point, the consultant was able to work with the group regarding the etiology of their prejudices—something like peeling an onion to get to the core. The goal was to rebuild it without taint—a task easier said than done in one session. But knowledge that a problem exists is a good start.

During the early days of AIDS care, it was controversial to admit AIDS patients to what we called scatter beds—empty beds on regular medical units. I was a CNE at the time and recall receiving an urgent message from a unit clerk stating that a maintenance employee would not enter a patient room to change a light bulb.

I went to the unit, and there, I found the worker standing stubbornly outside the door clutching his ladder. He was vigorously shaking his head refusing to go into the room despite the infectious disease (ID) nurse assuring him that he could not contract AIDS from a light bulb.

Upon arriving on the scene, the employee—in the presence of his union delegate and a gathering crowd—repeated his objection. I asked him if he planned to have sex with the patient. That brought him up short and speechless, which gave the ID nurse a chance to reinforce her teaching. At the end of her discourse, I took the ladder and entered the patient's room.

The maintenance worker followed me somewhat sheepishly and climbed the ladder, which I symbolically held in place. He deftly changed the bulb, took his ladder, and exited the room to a round of applause—including the patient's. The worker took a bow.

The morals of the story are severalfold: HIV/AIDS is a culture; cultures often clash; the best teaching is done by example; and a little humor goes a long way.

There are so many cultures that we in health care encounter—how can we possibly learn about them all? The short answer is—we cannot, but we can seek creative ways to learn some things.

CULTURE, RELIGION, AND THE FUNERAL CONNECTION

Culture, religion, and the way in which people deal with death—the way they conduct rituals surrounding death—all are vital components of the human condition. Knowledge of all three helps us meet our goals of providing patient-centered care. Of the many ways to learn about the myriad cultures and religions with which we come in contact, an unusual way is to attend funerals.

Simply attending a Catholic funeral mass, for example, will tell you a lot about how Catholics think and feel about an afterlife. That provides insight into how they might face serious illness and impending death, both as patients and as caregivers. This, of course, holds true for other religions as well.

Bear in mind that conflict will often arise with differences in religious beliefs, cultural mores and disparities in age, to name a few. There is only one constant and that is that there always are differences. This may sound elementary, but the truth is, it is extraordinarily complex. It illustrates the need for ongoing learning, cradle to grave.

Talking to all kinds of people can be an excellent source of information. Include clergy and lay people, professors, students, and philosophers. As we reviewed before, an important resource is Elisabeth Kübler-Ross's work, especially her seminal work—*On Death and Dying*. To gather her data, she used as her research team entry level staff among others.

In her work on death and dying, she describes five stages of grief: denial, anger, bargaining, depression, and acceptance.

I have found that the five stages of grief she describes extend beyond the dying—they extend to any major life event that presents a threat to the ego.

For example, You get a less than sterling performance appraisal and say—"No, I can't believe this." That is:

■ *Denial*
Then you get really mad at your supervisor. It is not your fault—it is hers! You did fine—she misperceived, or misunderstood, and that is pure and simple:
■ *Anger*
But soon you realize that neither denial nor anger is going to do you any good so you had better start thinking about a plan. What will do you good? Maybe if you promise to improve by a certain date. Maybe if you agree to write a report, or research a project, or . . . and that is:
■ *Bargaining*
But you start to wonder if that will work and maybe your supervisor will not accept your plan and maybe she will put you on notice and maybe. . . . You feel, sad, dejected, and worried that you will lose your job. You worry so much, it affects your sleep and your relationships and maybe even affects your job performance, and so you have reached the stage called:
■ *Depression*
But you are healthy, so eventually, you calm down and realize that it is up to you to do better—and that is:
■ *Acceptance*

These are all very important steps to help you maintain ego strength and leadership. As nurse managers, you have to set examples for your staff. One poor performance appraisal is not necessarily the end of the world *if* the culture of your organization is to assist, not punish. Is that what you do for your staff members? If you are a transformational leader—you do.

But for now, let us get back to our quest for knowledge; knowledge that will advance our understanding of the patients we care for and the multicultural staff we integrate into our team.

WHERE EAST MEETS WEST

In your quest for understanding, do not limit yourself to just the West. There is a vast store of information in the East, where the sun rises. Buddhism, Hinduism, Islam, Shinto, the Tao and more—millions of folks bend knee to many gods or to no god at all. This all influences how they live, think, act, and die; right here in America, we have Native Americans and their Shamanistic religions.

Human beings, in our egocentrism, go to the same church, synagogue, temple, shrine, or mosque—or not—all for most of our lives. It is familiar and comfortable. We study the tenets of our religion or do what the Good Book advises. The question is: How does that prepare us to care for patients of other cultures and religions at some of the most trying times of their lives—especially if we believe ours is the one true faith? Actually, it does not—unless we take the trouble to enlighten ourselves.

Comparative religion is not part of any nursing curriculum that I am aware of, but it is among the electives in most colleges and universities, and it is a fascinating subject. You may *feel* you have no time to add an elective to your busy day and that is understandable. But with the steady influx of immigrants into this country, we have no dearth of challenges in our health care settings. So think about how you can possibly provide holistic care to a multicultural patient mix without some understanding about their belief systems. For some suggestions as to *what* to read, check out a college curriculum for cross-cultural or multicultural studies or "do a Google" under similar subject headings.

STRANGERS IN A STRANGE LAND

Imagine traveling to, much less resettling in, a foreign land, becoming ill, ending up in a hospital, and not speaking the language. Terrifying is the first word that comes to my mind. So as not to face such a contingency, an ER nurse I knew, who loved to travel, prepared a travel medical bag complete with urinary catheters and IV equipment. He never left home without it.

But think of all the immigrants who resettle here in America. The good news for them is that Federal law requires informed consent prior to procedures being performed. This presupposes their comprehension. Comprehension presupposes the availability of interpretation of English into their language. That means that there must be interpreters readily available to meet patient needs. But it is impossible to cover *every* language—or is it? One would think properly programmed computers could meet this need. But do they?

So many questions. Would that there be answers to all these questions. Here is another question for you—one that is easier to answer. Should gender studies be included in family and community health education?

THE MAGIC KINGDOM OF HEALTH CARE

The need for family and community health education places it comfortably within nursing's realm. Gender studies also are an important issue in the nursing management and the clinical world, especially as it crosses cultural lines. Transgender and cross-gender issues affect all races, nationalities, and religions. These and related issues need to be discussed openly. Sweeping these sensitive matters under the rug only subverts the goal of patient-centered care. But there are so many ways to subvert that elusive goal of patient-centered care.

What follows is a story describing the decision-making process of a fiscal conservative comptroller that is not uncommon in the health care industry as has been experienced by and reported to this author. In the first case, cost-cutting without regard to patient-centered care prevailed. In the second case, both cost-cutting and patient-centered care were served.

Vignette   **Clash of the Titans**

The setting: Meeting of department heads of long-term care facility.
Chair: The administrator.
In attendance: Department heads of Medicine, Nursing, Therapies, Social Service, etc.
Agenda: Cost cutting. Points of agreement: personality types—all Type A.
And: No one could afford to cut even one position from their tables of organization (TO).
Rationale: To do so would compromise patient safety.
Time spent: One hour arguing.
Time remaining: All day.
Hope of reaching accord through conflict resolution methods discussed below: Unlikely.
Method ultimately chosen by administrator: Dictatorial.
He demanded that 10% be cut from the cumulative budget, and he did not care how. He then arose from his chair and headed for the door. Just before he left the room, he turned toward and told the group that they had 10 days in which to comply with his demand.

Whether or not conflict originates from transcultural issues or from other sources, differences and disagreements are almost constant companions and components of the human condition.

In the 1970s, Kenneth Thomas and Ralph Kilmann identified five main styles of dealing with conflict. They believed that individuals employ a characteristic conflict resolution technique. They also suggested that one style did not fit all encounters—much like situational leadership.

The Thomas–Kilmann Conflict Mode Instrument (TKI) is based on their findings and can assist an individual to recognize which style of conflict resolution she or he automatically selects when in a conflict situation. Not all are appropriate, however, when patient-centered care is the goal.

The Thomas and Kilmann's five conflict resolution behaviors are: competitive, collaborative, compromising, accommodating, and avoiding. Do you know which style feels natural to you? Let us take a look and start with the categories and characteristics as first promulgated by these two individuals.

Competitive: The competitor usually operates from a position of power that derives from rank, expertise, or persuasive ability. This is useful in emergencies and when rapid decisions are essential to saving life and limb. But competitive conduct can leave people feeling battered and distressed when applied in uncritical situations. So it is not an effective method to be applied by the existential manager over the long term when team building, motivation, and patient-centered care are the goals.

Collaborative: Collaborators try to meet everyone's needs. They may be extremely assertive, but unlike the competitor, they cooperate effectively. This style is valuable in bringing together many disparate perspectives to reach the best solution. However, collaborating takes time, and time may be short when problems exist that interfere with the three overarching goals mentioned above: team building, motivation, and patient-centered care.

Compromising: Compromisers try to satisfy everyone, at least to some degree. All participants are expected to relinquish something of equal value, including the compromiser. This is an effective method with impending deadlines, when the cost of divergence is greater than the cost of giving way, or when there is a stalemate. But beware—the thing relinquished may be just the thing needed to reach the ultimate goal.

Accommodating: The accommodator is highly cooperative, unassertive, and willing to meet the needs of others—often at personal expense. Warning! Resentment may develop if favors are not returned, and peace is not lasting. Peace, as history teaches us, is often impermanent.

Avoiding: Avoiders avoid. They will try almost anything to steer clear of conflict, including delaying and delegating controversial decisions, accepting previous and default decisions, and not wanting to hurt anyone's feelings. Avoiding does have its place for an interim or cooling off period, when the controversy is trivial, or when someone else is in a better position to solve the problem. Otherwise, avoidance in the face of conflict is a cop-out that interferes with patient-centered care.

Like situational leadership, the existential leader, working toward resolving conflict, should be able to draw on all these styles and apply them depending on the situation and the maturity level of the individuals involved in the situation. Style also depends on the situation itself. Just as with leader behavior styles, certain methods of conflict resolution feel better to one person than to another. But that does not mean you cannot learn to live with, and then master, all five approaches. The avoider can learn to compete, and the collaborator can learn to compromise.

Some of you may be thinking right about now: "When is avoidance a good thing?" The answer is, "It's a good thing when tempers flare, or when privacy is unavailable, or when other things take precedence."

Once the way has been cleared, you might discover that the problem has taken care of itself and conflict has been resolved—without your intervention. Remember, words and behaviors only have value based on context. For example, sometimes competition is good, and collaboration is bad. Competition may be good when it awakens people's ambitions, so they rise to levels of achievement even they did not think they could attain. Collaboration may be bad when the friend of my enemy collaborates against me, and the enemy of my enemy is my friend.

APIE . . . AND I DO NOT MEAN APPLE OR CHERRY

Here are another set of points to ponder. APIE in nursing has traditionally referred to the nursing process: Assess, Plan, Intervene, Evaluate. Remember that Florence Nightingale was celebrated for her assessment skills, and for the importance she placed on gathering statistics and transmitting her knowledge and her deep understanding of her patients to others assuming care. She knew, as we know today, responsibility cannot end when the nurse leaves the unit.

When shifts overlapped, face-to-face reports were one-on-one. If the incoming nurse had questions, she asked the outgoing nurse. Misunderstandings were immediately resolved.

Then, the culture changed. Shifts lost the overlap, and reports were written or audiotaped. Misunderstandings multiplied.

Computerization should effect positive change—where such technology exists and is correctly used. Nightingale knew then—and we of professional discernment know now—that the most professional assessment and treatment plan, even with elegant implementation, must be followed-up by evaluation then communicated to incoming caregivers. Otherwise, patient-centered care remains an elusive goal.

APIE as an Existential Management Device

As long as we have the nursing process to remind us of our professional strengths, why not apply it to our role as existential patient-centered leaders and managers? Many of us already do that as automatic reflexive acts. Now, let us examine the significance of what we do.

Assess the culture of the management environment. Is staff cooperative, or is there an undercurrent of hostility? Are they energetic or exhausted before they begin? Do they seem happy and pleased with their work, or anxious for their shift to end? Are there learning deficits?

Plan programs to comprehensively respond to the difficulties described above. Include a steering committee of involved staff members. Remember to bring in all levels of nursing staff and interdisciplinary staff as appropriate.

Implement those programs without diminishing patient-centered care. Obtain assistance from continuing education personnel, department of social services, psychology, and others. Consider infectious diseases and other resources available to you. Remember, you do not work in a vacuum.

Evaluate the effectiveness of this approach on your staff and patients. Remember to use all resources at your disposal—especially your own staff members. The more you include and empower them, the more they will grow into the roles you have helped them define. Effective communication, collaboration, team building, and patient-centered care will all improve.

Another factor to consider is the nursing process as a foundation of APIE from the phenomenological perspectives of Authenticity, Praxis, Idiosyncratic, and Existential.

Authenticity means being *true* to oneself, one's values, and one's beliefs—no matter the consequences. The exception: when one's beliefs are prejudiced against another's rights to be real and to be evaluated equally under the law, and under the condition of patient-centered care and respect for others.

Praxis—the act and art of applying theory to practice—comes after committing the time and effort necessary to learn, understand, abstract, articulate, and apply that *theoretical framework* to practice. Remember, this is a give and take relationship—like a delicate dance. First one, then the other: theory to practice, practice based on theory. . . . Both are strong and both are well balanced.

Idiosyncratic—what a truly boring world it would be if every person in it were like me. The point is that everyone is unique, individual, and different. It is those differences that are to be valued and nurtured.

Existential—the art of *being* in the world. Existentialism is a twentieth century philosophy that is complex in its entirety and its application. But like most things, it can be simplified. This is especially important for the purposes of understanding and application. From its very root, it is apparent that it has to do with (human) existence. So here is one of the less-convoluted definitions: Existentialism, according to Stewart and Mickunas,

> *is the insistence that human reality is situated in a concrete world-context. . . . man is only man as a result of his actions which are worked out in the world. The total ensemble of human actions—including thoughts, moods, efforts, emotions, and so forth—define the context in which man situates himself. But, in turn, the world-context defines and sets limits to human action.*

This leads us back to the issues of culture, which set limits in the world, and of cultural competence and cultural dissonance. That is a topic we are required by the Department of Health and Human Services to understand, so we can provide culturally competent care.

We need to appreciate what constitutes culture, how it differs from society, and where prejudice—anathema to a smoothly functioning society or to health care delivery—has its roots.

Culture includes activities, viewpoints, conduct, manners, facial expressions, values, religious beliefs, and objects that are common to a group or to a society. It is through a common culture that people share a language, customs, mores, values, rules, tools, organizations, and prejudices. It is through a mutual culture that individuals and groups define themselves. Example: I am Catholic. I conform to that society's shared values. I am pro-life and contribute to that society by, among other things, donating time and money to Catholic causes and to my local parish.

WHAT IS GOOD TO ONE IS BAD TO ANOTHER

Ours is a global culture of more than 6 billion people. We in health care, especially in our coastal cities, may be called upon to deliver culturally competent care—and to work with people whose mores, race, religious beliefs and practices are as different from ours as is day from night. So too, are common behaviors and communication patterns and reactions to everyday occurrences. That includes such mundane things as pain, dietary restrictions, and taste in food. What is good to one culture may be terrible to another.

The question is, how do we differentiate good from bad when it comes to the human being? The answer is obvious in its simplicity—we do not. Only the individual culture can do that.

Fact or Fiction—You Decide

I overheard an argument the other day between two men—one from Puerto Rico and the other from the Dominican Republic. The gist of the conversation was the accusation that Dominicans are jealous of Puerto Ricans because Puerto Ricans have privileges of American citizenship and Dominicans do not.

Next, I heard that Hispanics care for their elderly, while Jews—who have fewer children, as a rule—do not. They place their parents in nursing homes instead. The retort was that the first group has so many children that they have enough individuals in the family to care for their aged. The response to that was that they are in public-subsidized housing—on welfare—while Jews are self-sustaining, obviously wild prejudice-based allegations. Neither offered any support for their point of view. Human beings often act on what they *feel* and not necessarily on what they *know*. Factual data do not seem to matter.

Here is another example of faulty statistics. A cab driver recently turned to me and said: "Are you a Jew?" When I responded "Yes," he proceeded to tell me that he was a Muslim from Pakistan and that he had an 80% probability of being murdered if he went to Israel. He could not cite his source, nor could he be swayed from his belief.

Points in fact: According to the Israeli Foreign Ministry, 2009 statistics, 18% to 20% of Israeli citizens are Arabic speaking. Some are Christian, some are Druze, and some are Muslim. Although I diligently searched, I could find no significant murder statistics for Muslim citizens or visitors in Israel.

An African American colleague of mine—a well-educated and doctorally prepared nurse educator—insisted that my Jewish ancestors owned slave ships that brought her ancestors here from Africa. Doubly appalled, once for the practice of slavery and secondly that she would make such an assertion, I asked for her source of information. "Everyone knows," she replied.

Points in fact: My ancestors could not have owned slave ships—they came from Eastern Europe, and many of them never made it out of Russia. They were either killed in the Tsar's Pogroms or by the Nazis during World War II.

The Governor of Texas recently called for secession of his state. Does he not know that secessionism is an anti-black theme from Civil War days—and that this is highly prejudicial against African Americans?

In the rural, urban, and suburban areas of our beloved country lurk bigots of every stripe and color. There are anti just about everything. Some are well aware of their prejudices, and others believe it is the norm because they were *carefully taught* to believe what they believe.

In the Rodgers and Hammerstein show *South Pacific*, there is the following song that perfectly illustrates this point:

You've Got To Be Carefully Taught
by
Richard Rodgers & Oscar Hammerstein II

You've got to be taught to hate and fear,
You've got to be taught from year to year,
It's got to be drummed in your dear little ear—
You've got to be carefully taught.

You've got to be taught to be afraid
Of people whose eyes are oddly made,
And people whose skin is a different shade—
You've got to be carefully taught.

You've got to be taught before it's too late,
Before you are six or seven or eight,
To hate all the people your relatives hate—
You've got to be carefully taught!
You've got to be carefully taught!

Vignette   She Had Been Carefully Taught—But So Was I

When I was a little girl, I came home from school one day and found our housekeeper, Mae—a Southern black woman—lying on the floor in the bathroom.
"Why are you here, Mae?" I asked.
"Because I'm sick," she replied.
"Why didn't you go to bed?" I asked.
"Because I can't lie in no white person's bed," she answered.
"Yes you can." I said as I helped her get up from the floor and into my mother's bed. I then called the doctor.
You see, *I* had been carefully taught.

MAKING A LIST AND CHECKING IT TWICE

So, how do we take deep-seated prejudices that have been carefully taught while we were growing up, and override them as adults? The answer is simple in its construction but extremely difficult in its application. Start with the easy part: First, acknowledge that these prejudices exist by listing everything you dislike or hate. Just write down whatever comes to your mind. Do not think too much about what you write. Make it an off-the-cuff list.

Here is a list of things I actually heard from someone I know:

He hated Jews, New Yorkers, Italians, fat people, African Americans, Puerto Ricans and other Hispanics, and all immigrants—except from Ireland. He also hated outspoken women, bleached blondes, flat-chested women and a score of others.

This might have been funny, since he was Catholic and often talked of having been the butt of prejudice himself while growing up in a Midwest Protestant community where he was often called fish-eater or mackerel-snapper as he was smacked around by kids larger than he. But would it still be amusing if he had had the power to hire or fire, or to give or withhold care, to be a little rough?

Where do you suppose all those bruises come from that blossom on the fragile arms of the elderly in nursing homes and in hospitals? Why all the pressure injuries—decubiti in our patient units? Not exactly patient-centered care as you or I might define it, is it? Might some of these iatrogenic conditions be the result of suppressed prejudice?

Prejudice is a dangerous thing. Read the history of any genocidal effort—13 million dead at the hands of the Nazis. Six million of them were Jews, many of whom died as a direct or indirect result of the duplicity of friends and neighbors. One day, they were playing soccer together, and the next, they were herded into death camps or shot dead as they stood naked on the rim of trenches already fetid with the stench of corpses.

Nicholas Kristoff, a columnist for the *New York Times*, often bears witness to the horrors of genocidal murder as well as the rapes of children in the Congo, while the world looks on. There recently were Congressional hearings about Armenians in Turkey. Was it or was it not a genocidal effort? Darfur, Chechnya, Rwanda, the list goes on as it has throughout history. But these places are far away. Bring the issue of prejudice into your own backyard.

Is your list of personal prejudices yet prepared? Now analyze the etiology of those feelings. What was the source? Did you hear it at your dinner table or in your school playground? How about at the grocery store or at the movies? It really does not matter *where* you heard it, but how old you were and how many times and how much influence the bigot had over you. The fact is the hatred has become ingrained in you, and you must scrub it out with the same persistence you have put into other important things. Here is how to start.

Make it a point to place yourself in the presence of that which you hate. Is it African Americans, Haitians, Hispanic immigrants, or Orthodox Jews? First, write down why you hate them. Then, volunteer your services where they are in large numbers—English as a second language center or a Hispanic health clinic, for example. Get to know some immigrants as individuals. You will likely be surprised as you discover the many endearing qualities of the people you thought were monstrous.

Translate this knowledge to patient-centered care. Remember the walk-a-mile-in-my-shoes imperative. As a nurse manager, you are responsible for pulling together a patient-centered team, and like Joseph's dream coat of many colors, your team members may resemble a tapestry of many hues, so start embroidering.

You can apply this concept to any group you have identified. Just do not sweep anything under the rug. It will come back to haunt you and worse. It will negatively impact members of your team and then your ability to guarantee effective patient-centered care.

Think about the ethnic groups with whom you have regular contact. These are the people you need to know. Consider them from a multicultural perspective and in your management role or patient-centered care relationships. But *before* you make eye contact, shake someone's hand, or offer a wink, a nod, or a smile, better think again.

The July 13th, 2009 edition of *Nursing Spectrum*'s continuing education program, by Kathleen D. Pagana, PhD, RN, entitled, "Mind Your Manners. . . . Multiculturally" is a handy reference upon which the existential manager may rely when culturally competent communication is required among and between staff and patients. Some of the aforementioned gestures just might be misunderstood. There are others. Putting your hands on your hips is innocuous to an American, but this may be viewed as an aggressive challenge to someone from Mexico or Argentina. And think what effect it might have in an adolescent psych unit, for example.

A simple "thumbs up" in America—frequently used to encourage someone—is rude throughout the Arab world. That wink Sarah Palin made famous is a big no-no in Australia, Taiwan, and other countries, according to Pagana.

There is more. All of it is as intriguing as it is important to both sides of the communication dyad—you and the other person. If there are many people surrounding the patient, or supporting the staff member as in a union situation, it helps the existential manager to have her multicultural ducks in a row. At least she will not make the *faux pas* of looking someone in the eye who, by cultural norms, maintains an averted, sidelong glance.

But there are many more pitfalls one can trip into in the health care milieu. It is important, therefore, to know what yours in particular are. See the figure entitled *sensitivity training* at the end of this chapter for suggestions on how to tailor a program to your particular needs. Doing so broadcasts the existential manager's goal to create an empathetic, fair management environment in which staff and patients *feel* accepted for their differences as well as for their similarities.

A LAND OF HOPE AND GLORY

America has not only been a tourist destination, it has also been a "land of hope and glory" for literally millions of immigrants coming from distant lands. They are seeking—and often find—a better life. They bring with them their native tongue, dress, culture, and religion as they practiced it from birth, and a host of other things that are often strange to their new neighbors.

History teaches us that first-generation immigrants often do not assimilate easily, if at all. They frequently retain their native tongues, food choices, and customs. But they often encourage their children to embrace the ways of their new home.

But what about nurses who have been educated elsewhere and who come here to work—sometimes one, sometimes in groups of two, three, four or more? Do they incorporate the larger culture more easily? Or do they congregate together, sharing a common language and idiom of speech, dress, and food choice? Let us take a look.

Nursing Shortages—A Recurring Theme

Nursing shortages are cyclical. They are a persistent recurrence in the history of American health care. During times of war, when RNs are diverted to military service at home and abroad, these shortages are especially troubling. American health care organizations have turned time and again to importing nurses from abroad. This creates several sets of problems, two of which stand out from among the rest:

- The moral dilemma that flows from enticing nurses to leave their countries already strapped by nursing shortages of their own to come here for the promise of better salaries and benefits.
- The cultural dissonance caused by intermingling large groups of foreign nurses sometimes with smaller groups of American nurses.

Vignette   They Knew, But Knowing Is Not Doing

Her name was Angie. She was a white, American-born Catholic of Italian ancestry and had been employed as a registered nurse into a staff level position by the hospital 4 years previous to her filing her complaint. Her performance, attendance, and other parameters of employment were without blemish.

Wanting to advance her career, she had enrolled in a master's program at a local university, completed the management development course offered by the hospital, and applied for promotion. Each time a position became available, she was skipped over and someone with less seniority was promoted instead. This was a union-free environment, so she filed complaints each time with her supervisor, the human resources director, and her CNE. She contended that her requests were being ignored due to favoritism based on nationality. This took place during a time when large groups of nurses had been recruited from abroad during an acute nursing shortage. Cliques were not uncommon, and groups of foreign nurses often gathered together and spoke their native language on the nursing units. Cultural dissonance, isolation, and hard feelings resulted.

In Angela's case, it was unfortunate that her CNE failed to assist her. Her story came to me through a colleague who was visiting her sick mother in Angela's hospital. She counseled Angela to gather her facts and once again seek assistance from her hierarchy and then from human resources. If the individuals within her work environment failed to intervene on her behalf, she was advised to contact the Human Rights Commission.

Management is responsible for stopping such practices. Favoritism as a parameter for promotion and cliques that keep outsiders out interfere with patient-centered care. To ignore this is to interfere with the very practices that we are committed to support—building and sustaining relationships that benefit staff and patients.

Culturally competent care relies on effective communication. In this polyglot world, we must make a choice. Since this is the United States, we must choose English as the primary language. Of course, there always are exceptions.

Vignette   Don't Be a Fool—Break the Rules

The Place: a nursing unit in a large university-affiliated teaching medical center. The facility has a long-standing policy prohibiting employees from speaking languages other than English in public places—except when communicating to patients or significant others as appropriate.

The Circumstance: A nursing supervisor overhears a unit secretary speaking Spanish into a telephone at a nursing station. The supervisor interrupts the employee, tells her to end the conversation and accompany her to her office where she reprimands her and issues a suspension without asking for or listening to an explanation. She later learns that the employee had received an emergency telephone call from her non-English speaking mother, informing her that her father had suddenly died.

Discussion: There are so many things wrong with this scenario I hardly know where to begin. First, there should always be exceptions to every rule—you simply cannot think of everything when you are writing policy. In most union contracts, there is a management's rights clause stating: all other duties and responsibilities as assigned by management. This is a catch-all phrase because no one should be expected to think of everything at the time they are promulgating a contract—or a policy, for that matter. Add this caveat, or you will wish you had when it is too late.

The next problem with the above example should have hit you by now—you have probably heard it before. *Act in haste, repent in leisure.*

The supervisor was not facing an emergency. There was no need for alacrity. Nothing was to be gained by rushing the employee off the phone.

Had the supervisor bothered to find out what caused the employee to break the rules, she might have offered sympathy instead of reprimand. She might have looked like a hero instead of a fool.

This scenario is very different from the daily events in which groups of coworkers speak to each other in their native language while on duty. No matter what the personnel policies state—when out of earshot of a supervisor—they often revert to old habits. Wouldn't you? Many of their patients speak that same language, but it is *okay* for them to use it—right? So, what is the existential manager to do?

Be sensible, level-headed, sane, rational, and wise. In my perfect world, I would get the policy that demands that everyone speak English off the books and write a policy that is *provisional*. It is like the economics professor's advice—*it depends.*

Before I get to my suggestions for a sensitivity training survey, I want to open a can of worms—or a many-faceted problem. A newly admitted patient or patient's family asks to see you. Maybe they are white—or black. Maybe they are Muslim or Jewish. Maybe they are straight or gay. It does not really matter what they are, it matters what they request. Let us say, for example, that a white family asks that only a white staff member care for their mother. What do you do?

Let us assume you are white. But what if you are black? Is your temper rising? I would not blame you if it were, but that will not help you deal with the problem. What you can do is as follows:

- You can revert to policy—"policy prohibits us from making assignments according to race or religion"—and deal with an irate family.
- You can agree, assign a white staff member and take on an irate staff while trying to explain your decision.
- You can inquire as to why such a request is being made and use your professional, empathetic, phenomenological intelligence to respond accordingly. Maybe there is a good reason for this request— or maybe it is pure hatred.
- You can duck the issue and say you will get back to them while you seek counsel from your supervisor or others.

There are many avenues open to you. What you should *not* do is react emotionally to what appears to be a no-way-out situation. And while we are on the subject of emotional reactiveness, let us discuss this all too common human response.

Do you blush? Do you get hot under the collar? Does your temper rise? Have you studied visceral reactions? Most people will give away their feelings through physiological responses over which they have little control—and that means you will, too. So when you are dealing with someone you do not like—keep it cerebral if you can. If you cannot, a time out might be in order. Remember, the only real emergencies involve fire, cardiac arrests, and other life-threatening events. Most other things will not suffer from a hiatus of time—in fact, they might benefit.

Here's an example:

Vignette   We Will Care Only for Our Own

It was in the midst of a major job action. All support service staff were out on picket lines. A large number of debilitated nursing home patents required feeding and attendant care—three meals a day for what turned out to be more than 3 weeks. A local religious school offered to send its students, parents, and teachers three times a day for the duration of the strike to help feed and care for the patients. But they would only attend to those of their faith.

With fear and trepidation the director of patient care services told the religious leader that unless they would minister to all patients identified by the professionals at the facility as needing care, their offer would have to be declined.

Hours went by during which emergency plans were made to transfer patients who needed complete care due to varying degrees of severe dementia and Alzheimer's disease. A transfer would certainly disorient them more.

At the 11th hour, the religious leader relented, and busloads of teenagers and teachers arrived, thus alleviating the need for transfer. Their services were invaluable to the patients, and I daresay also to the volunteers. Their decision to break the religious and cultural barriers that they themselves had imposed had to go a long way to realign their thinking. At the very least, they exposed their young people—who had been secluded from a secular world—to the fact that people different from themselves were really similar in so many ways.

These volunteers had trouble getting across a rowdy and sometimes violent picket line but that did not stop them. They formed tight V-shaped wedges and broke through the blockades three times a day, every day for the duration of the strike. After all, their patients needed them—white, black, Jewish, Christian. After the first self-imposed obstacle was crossed, the only one left was that which the picketers created.

FOOTNOTE: SENSITIVITY TRAINING

This is about management's obligation to provide staff with formalized cultural diversity training. Here are some questions:

- Should management bring in an official training company?
- Should it be a generic training program?
- Should it be from an academic or psychological perspective?
- What cultures should be included?

There seem to be a number of *shoulds* in the above list. But no matter how many *shoulds* are covered in the program, there will be a number of *coulds* left over. For example, someone might say, "They *could* have covered things like the culture of being younger than everyone else—or older." Or, "They *could* have covered fat people or people who are too thin."

After all, it is not just race and religion that are cultural outliers. People pick on one another because of many other kinds of personality and physical traits.

Unless you fit your programs to your organization's demographics, you will likely be out on a limb. Consider sensitivity training individualized to your staff and patient population and think about making it in-depth and didactic. Be careful to include the nondominant cultures, even if you are tempted not to. Remember, even small problems can lead to negative and nasty outcomes.

Be sure to include both your patient population and your staff. Prepare confidential, written surveys. But conduct private interviews with your patients. See Exhibit 6.1 for a sample.

EXHIBIT 6.1 | CULTURAL SENSITIVITY SURVEY

Dear Staff Member:

Management is conducting a sensitivity survey to see how you feel about working here. Please answer as frankly as possible. All responses will be kept strictly confidential. There is no identifying information on this form. Your replies will be used to develop sensitivity training for management and staff. It is our goal to improve your work environment.

Please insert the completed form into envelopes provided within 2 weeks. Seal and drop the envelope into the box marked *Sensitivity Survey* near the time clocks. Once results are collated, we will publish a report in the next newsletter.

Thank you.

1. Do you *feel* you have ever been treated unfairly because of your *race, religion, national origin, sexual orientation, age, physical appearance, speech patterns, education, licensure, certification, job title,* other? Please *CIRCLE* all that apply and *ADD COMMENTS*:

   _____
   _____
   _____
   _____

2. Do you believe you have ever been denied requests for promotion, transfer, change of assignment, holiday, vacation, overtime etc., because of any of the above?
   YES ___ NO ___ Please *CIRCLE* all that apply and
   ADD COMMENTS _____

   _____

   _____
   _____

3. I am Male _____ Female _____
4. I have been employed here _____ years
5. I am _____ years old
6. I am: white _____ hispanic _____
   African _____ Specify _____
   African American _____
   Caribbean_____
   Asian _____ Specify _____
   Pacific Islander _____ Specify _____
   Other _____
7. Staff Title _____ License _____
   Comments_____

   _____

   _____
   _____

                                            Thank you!

Now you can adapt your programs based on actual data you have collected. You will know if staff and management have minimized problems, or if problems have been minimal. If you have also interviewed patients, you will have a full range of data. This is a cost-effective way to bridge the cultural divide, increase sensitivity, and encourage team building—all important in the ongoing quest for patient-centered care.

SUMMARY

This chapter examines issues, and similarities and differences of culture, religion, prejudice, race, mores, and habits that dictate behavior and influence human thinking and behavior from cradle to grave.

- Existentialism—human reality is situated in a concrete world context—man is only man as a result of his actions worked out in the world (Stewart and Mikunas, 1990).
- Culture—activities, viewpoints, objects, manners, facial expressions, and more set limits and define cultural competence, and cultural dissonance characterize things that may be good to one culture but bad to another.
- Cultural dissonance that exists in health care delivery organizations interfere with patent-centered care.
- Deep-seated prejudice—origins, effects, amelioration. Prejudicial ideas and excuses influence action.
- Conflict resolution and the use of the nursing process to improve management culture—Use of humor to ease tensions.
- Conflict Resolution Styles (Thomas and Killman) are like Leader Behavior Styles—choose the style appropriate to the situation.
- Multilingualism: Should we have policies against languages other than English being spoken on nursing units? The answer, as it is so often, is: It depends.
- Cultural Sensitivity Survey: Helps you gather information to adapt your programs based on actual data.
- You will know if staff and management have minimized problems, or problems have been minimal.

CHAPTER ENDNOTES

Department of Health and Human Services. (FR Doc. 00-32685filed 12-21-00).

Rodgers, R., and O. Hammerstein, II. *You've got to be carefully taught*. New York: Williamson Music, 1949.

Stewart, D. and A. Mickunas. 1990. *Exploring phenomenology*, 2nd ed. Athens, OH: Ohio University Press.

Thomas, K. W. and R. H. Killman. Conflict Mode Instrument (TKI) Mountain View, CA: CPP, Inc. 1974–2009. http://www.kilmann.com/conflict.html (Accessed May 18, 2010).

7

Spirituality and Nursing: Challenges, Dilemmas, and Occasional Successes

Barbara Stevens Barnum, RN, PhD, FAAN

This book is strong on teaching by vignettes from experience, so true to the instinct of the author, Dr. Forman, I am going to try the same method. I am not even going to worry about defining *spirituality* until we emerge from our beginning example, which concerns nursing and spirituality.

The first vignette concerns the death of a cancer patient in a hospital/ hospice dedicated to terminal patient care. The majority of their patients are terminal cancer cases. The leadership in this institution—administrative, nursing, physician staff, and chaplaincy staff—work under the same set of specified values. Although these value statements are well publicized, one could not logically expect all patients' families to understand them with any subtlety, especially at the time a beloved relative is dying. These values were always shared with patients and their families. This institution went overboard to help people understand their value system.

In this vignette, a family threatened to sue because their loved one, the father of four adult siblings, died of an *overdose* of morphine. The hospital countered this threat by explaining what was carefully written in their literature and truly dominated their belief system: that their chief objective was pain relief for dying patients, and that, if a patient died from pain relief, the respiratory interference that caused death would be seen as a side effect; unwanted, but a side effect of pain relief nonetheless. The staff reminded these grown children that their policies and goals had been discussed in depth at the time of the patient's arrival 2 weeks earlier (with the two siblings who were then present). The mother of these adult siblings was long since deceased.

These policies allowed the institution's staff to claim (and believe) that they did not support euthanasia. The patients in this institution really did die *better* (more comfortable) deaths than patients in most other places. The patients' comfort was considered above all else. This family, however, chose to see the family member's death otherwise.

This situation was rife with elements related to spirituality. It was clear that the family members were in deep grief, yet they seemed to lack any religious or philosophic beliefs that might have given them comfort. Despite the fact that they knew their father had come to this place to die, as so often happens, the *facts* were in conflict with the *feelings*. Yes, they knew their father was dying, but that did not mean they had accepted the imminent death at a deep spiritual level. This was especially true of the two siblings who arrived from out of state during the very last week of the father's life.

The staff believed that some of the family members had unresolved issues with the father and that these feelings were the real underpinning beneath the threat of a lawsuit. One sign of their discomfort with even the thought of death was that the siblings were not able to discuss his coming death with their father. When he tried to bring up the subject, they used statements of denial, like, "Not so, Dad, you're going to get better." The staff was not able to crack through these defense mechanisms, but they were also limited by the short time in which the father was hospitalized (just under two full weeks).

Could the family have been better prepared if the father lived longer, if the staff (nurses, physicians, chaplains) had more time for family counseling? But it was not to be: the father died after his second week of admission.

The siblings' response was to lash out with the threat of a lawsuit. In this sense, the case also entered the domain of ethics—out of the realm of feelings, into the realm of adjudication.

The case was ultimately settled before it went to court, but it could easily have gone the other direction. In addition to the problems instigated by what appeared to be unfinished parent/child agendas, this confrontation illustrated the clash of well-intentioned value systems. Values are subtle, but they play out in very specific actions. Even persons who appear to lack a supportive belief structure (like these adult siblings), still ultimately hold some values as most meaningful in life.

In the above case, one could play the ethics game and note that the hospital staff centered its values in *intentions*, while the family centered their values in *effects*. Was it the *effect* of giving morphine that was the ethical criterion? Or the *intention* behind giving it that mattered? Which was the more important criterion?

One could spend hours arguing about which criterion was the appropriate one in evaluating what happened. Indeed, if one studied the case like a scholar, one could add other potential criteria like: God's word or the rules of a given religion.

Questions like this take us into the domain of *ethics* and philosophic debate. Ethics is the label given to the study of right and wrong. Yes, ethics deal with matters of spirituality, but in a peculiar way, the spiritual elements can almost get lost in the weighing of rights and wrongs.

Indeed, in this case, the staff was convinced that the protest about the father's death as an effect of morphine was not the real issue. The real issues, claimed the staff, were the unresolved feelings the children held concerning their father and concerning death itself. But it was simpler for the siblings to externalize and shift their claims to issues of ethics rather than deal with them as issues of personal feelings.

This case serves to illustrate that it is not always easy to separate issues of spirituality and ethics. But when the family responded by threatening legal action, it essentially became a case ruled by form, by ethics: What was right? What was wrong? The *intention* (pain relief) or the *effect* (death)?

If we want to differentiate between ethics and spirituality, we might make a simplistic separation by saying that ethics takes place mostly in the left brain, the logical thinking brain, while spirituality takes place mostly in the right brain, the feeling brain. Yes, of course, there are crossovers, but ethics mostly has to do with reasoning, while spirituality has to do with matters of the heart.

It is difficult to say just what *spirituality* involves. For some, that term is equivalent to *religion*; for others, these terms are not the same. Still, others would argue that they are very spiritual while holding no religion at all. Yet others equate spirituality with a broad humanism. Spirituality defies definition, but always it resides in the person's most important values, those truly held whether or not they are verbally espoused. These are the values that underlie the most important decisions that one makes in life, the values that affect one's actions. Spirituality involves the feelings one has about the things that matter most in life. In other words, it is what underlies the person's most intimate and intense sense of meaning.

Ethics is so much simpler than spirituality. Almost every profession has a code of ethics; nursing is no exception. Indeed, we have a code published by the American Nurses' Association (*Code of Ethics With Interpretive Statement*, 2001). But codes of ethics are forms of *to do* lists: they tell you what to do (in general terms) but not what to feel. Even in their directive function, such lists typically fail to tell you what to do when the circumstances are in any way unique—which seems to be more often than not. Even the ANA's *Code of ethics* cannot give protocols for every imagined situation.

Helpful as they may be, neither codes, philosophies, nor humanitarian principles can ultimately place an absolute judgment on actions. There are always grounds for interpretation—so many grounds.

If the vignette of the dying relative illustrates a mixed spiritual and ethical crisis, let us move to an even more difficult place.

Here is a vignette to illustrate the complexity of assessing spirituality. This situation occurred in a step-down unit to which a patient had just been transferred from an intensive care unit. A new young nurse, let us call her Lillian, was attempting to perform a nursing diagnosis for this patient whose care had been assigned to her. (We will take the liberty of using her first name because that was the way she introduced herself to the patient.)

Using a nursing diagnostic format, she asked the patient about his faith, noting that he was listed as holding one of the Judeo-Christian religions, although not the one to which she herself belonged.

The patient said, "Yeah, I listed that when I checked in before surgery, but I don't really believe in it. It doesn't make sense when you really look at it. The religion says a lot of things that contradict each other. And why should I keep a religion just because my parents believe it? They're no geniuses. I have some real doubts about it, to be honest."

The conversation went on in this fashion until the patient said, "Look I don't want to talk about this." But that did not stop Lillian from coming back to the subject time after time. After all, she was concerned with the diagnosis she had given him: spiritual distress.

This was a very important diagnosis for Lillian, as she was, in her own notion of self, a very *spiritual* person, heavily involved in her religious faith. Even though the patient was from another faith, she thought that, through her conversations, she might get him to drop his doubts and renew his religious commitment.

What she failed to recognize was that the patient was becoming more and more uncomfortable by her constant return to the subject of religion (her interpretation of spirituality). He even wondered if she might be trying to woo him to her own faith. Eventually, he became so uncomfortable that he asked that this nurse be removed from his care. He felt that he had enough to do in coping with his physical recovery.

His request upset Lillian greatly. As she saw it, she was only trying to treat a valid nursing diagnosis: spiritual distress.

Let us look at this vignette for a moment—and the challenges it presented to the nurse leader, in this case, the head nurse. In many ways, Lillian was performing on a high level, given her relatively recent graduation.

She was attempting to substantiate her practice with a cognitive basis, that is, the use of nursing diagnoses, and she was, on the whole, a very motivated nurse.

Yet, if we apply a *measure* of spirituality to the patient's and nurse's behaviors, we find an interesting contrast. Let us use M. Scott Peck's stages of spiritual growth (*Further Along the Road Less Traveled*, 1993). His first stage is characterized by an absence of spirituality, with unprincipled and manipulative behavior. Clearly, this stage has nothing to do with our case.

Stage two in Peck's theory involves formal/institutional faith, submission to rules of some code, most often found in an organized religion. According to Peck's descriptions, Lillian could be diagnosed as ranking at stage two. Her spirituality was best represented by her religion. The symbols and rituals of this nurse's religion were deeply tied to her notion of spirituality.

Peck's stage three involves questioning, seeking, shifting from unthinking submission to a state of deep truth-seeking about meaning. Indeed, when we look at the patient's behavior, he would be classified at stage three—a deeper stage than Lillian's, but often seen as rebellious and negative when viewed from stage two vision. But stage three evinces the first real exploring of spiritual values.

Peck's fourth stage deals with mystical vision, seeing beneath the surface of things—a stage of faith usually for saints and sages. This stage clearly was not applicable in our vignette to either Lillian or the patient.

In our case, Lillian's arguments to the patient were cast, naturally, at her level of faith. After all, that is where she was, and from there, she diagnosed the patient as in spiritual distress. Her idealized solution would have been for him to return to stage two, to once again accept his original faith and find solace in it.

The same dynamic would have happened on almost any developmental spiritual theory (and there are many). Take James Fowler's classic Stages of Faith (*Stages of Faith*, 1981). This tool would have classified Lillian at a stage that usually begins in adolescence, is characterized by acceptance of a normative value system in which the authority is external to the self. The holder of this belief stage can articulate the accepted faith, defend it, and feel deep emotions concerning it. Yet that faith is not an object of reflection. Indeed, the fact that its origin is external to the self discourages such reflection. Notice how closely this description resembles Peck's stage two.

Similarly, Fowler would have placed the patient on a higher level than Lillian, a phase where the authority for spirituality is brought back into the self, and a system of faith is actually examined by the person. It is not unusual for persons at this level of spiritual (or religious) inquiry to lose faith in the system that was the source of their earlier faith. Fowler's stage described above, much like Peck's stage three, would have placed the patient in this phase; that is, one step more advanced than his nurse.

Yet the very traits that marked the patient's new level of spiritual growth were assessed by Lillian (herself at a lower level) as failures. There was no way this nurse could see, from her level of spiritual development, that the patient was at a higher level. It would be like asking a first grader to understand algebra.

Ironically, one can find this same unidimensional notion of spirituality in the North American Nursing Diagnosis Association's discussion of spiritual distress. Questioning of faith is labeled by NANDA as a negative situation. Keeping to one's original spirituality level (in our example, at Peck's level two) would be labeled as good. For the patient to return to this state would be seen as the optimal solution.

Hence, sadly, one of our own organizations sees faith as a stable state of *being*, not a state allowing for deeper and deeper development or, as a philosopher might say, a state of being versus a state of becoming.

Using Peck's theory (or numerous other spiritual theories that involve development of faith), the nursing judgment that the patient should be returned to his original spiritual state is ironic because life traumas, including illnesses, are often the impetus for an individual to begin to move to a higher conceptualization of spirituality.

So that, irreverently, one might be tempted to say, "He's upset and in doubt? Good for him; he's growing spiritually!" To nurses making judgments about a field in which they have little education, this might seem like an insane interpretation. Yet one could argue that, if the patient's jaded view of his past religious acceptances were stirred by his health situation, on Peck's scales, that would be the beginning development of an ultimately deeper faith.

In contrast, the nursing diagnosis of spiritual distress assumes that any judgments on this diagnosis are unidimensional: there simply is faith or no faith. No subtleties allowed please. Questioning past beliefs causes spiritual distress. That is all there is to that.

In this particular vignette, the head nurse felt herself to be in a real dilemma. She believed that she had to honor the patient's request, even though she knew it would make Lillian feel terrible. Ultimately, the head nurse simply removed Lillian from this patient's care and cautioned her against taking this route of discussion with other patients.

From the patient's perspective the problem was solved. From Lillian's perspective, she was left in a state of angst, convinced that the head nurse failed to understand the importance of spiritual distress. (Indeed, one might say at this stage Lillian felt she had her own case of spiritual distress.) Additionally, she felt humiliated by her first admonition from an authority figure.

The nurse leader felt bad about Lillian, yet did not know what else she might have done. Had the head nurse greater depth in spirituality herself—or greater knowledge about it as a subject matter—she might have handled the situation in a different manner. Assuming she knew anything about the literature and research on spirituality, could she have taken Lillian aside and given her a crash course in levels of spirituality? But could such enhanced knowledge actually speed up the maturing of the young nurse's faith?

This is what makes spirituality a teacher's nightmare. Yes, content can be given, and it can be very helpful to the person struggling with spiritual values. But content alone does not determine one's level of spiritual development.

If it truly is a matter that requires a certain level of life experience and maturity, as many claim, it would be unrealistic to expect Lillian to change her orientation because of something the head nurse taught (*content*). Might any such interference by the head nurse not be the same as demanding that a teenager act like an adult?

I think that different stages of faith often are at the bottom of the problems in which staff and patients clash or, indeed, problems where staff members disagree with each other. Yet, it also is true that the head nurse might have said something that stayed in Lillian's mind, only to come back to her consciousness years later when she might be struggling with her own developing spiritual maturity.

Content is important, but does not, by itself, create or alter the depth of one's spirituality. Spirituality is one of those things that must be internalized, that must become a part of the person's very being. Impetus for spiritual change seldom resides solely in a lecture.

In essence, to deal seriously with states of spirituality is helped by knowledge of the subject that most nurses simply lack. Yet knowledge alone is not an answer.

This is not a new pattern; indeed, it is a pattern that haunts nursing care. By the very fact of *being there*, nurses come to include many things in their notion of work that they were not educated to do. As nursing grows more technical in many ways, this complexity is not eliminated. Nurses are *there* with patients when things happen.

Issues of spirituality, like many other facets of care, may arise in situations for which the nurse is ill prepared. So we are thrust back on the question of whether the nurse acts or calls desperately for someone else who may or may not be available (a chaplain, for example) for what she perceives as needed spiritual care. Hence, the same old dilemma: the existential necessity for nurses to deal with phenomena for which they have little or no professional education, despite the fact that they are often the only ones present in the situation.

To make things even more complex, spirituality is a very personal thing. At least in our society, there is no demand that we all march to the same spiritual drummer. How then can one expect to educate nurses about spirituality and inculcate appropriate spiritual responses in nurses, knowing that no two people are the same? It is a daunting task and probably the reason why spirituality appears in so few curricula. If, however, spirituality is merely *assumed* to be an aspect of every nurse's psyche, what can we expect of them? Is it logical to anticipate a relatively high stage of spiritual maturity in all our nurses? Or is that unrealistic?

Older nurses may be more mature about it; they have experienced pain, loss, death, and faced tough situations in their own personal lives. If a high level of spirituality is typically (although not necessarily) associated with other measures of maturing, must we take that into consideration? The profession can hardly decide not to accept students, let us say, under 40 years of age. Practicalities reign. Logic dictates that we will educate nurses who hold various degrees of spiritual development, as well as hold wide differences in their spiritual values.

Is it enough to make nurses aware of some of the cultural and behavioral aspects attached to various common religions? Is it enough that the nurse learns simply to respect these differences? Is it enough, in other words, that the nurse learns a few processes and a few general dictates (respect for the beliefs of others, respect for religious dietary demands, etc.)? Is it enough that the nurse upholds what we might better label as humanistic values rather than what might be termed spiritual values? Is it enough to give her a code of ethical behavior?

Most professions have certain covert expectations for its members— things that arise in the context of practice more than in content presented. In nursing, the covert requirement of some level of what we might label spiritual competency has waxed and waned over the years. For many decades now, nursing has focused on proving itself as a worthy academic discipline. In essence, this has shifted nursing from espousing its spiritual roots to advocating its scientific underpinnings.

This shift is often indicated in the writings about Florence Nightingale. I think of the book by Dossey et al., (*Florence Nightingale Today: Healing, Leadership, Global Action*, 2005) as the best example of a balanced view of Nightingale. But this book is the exception. At one time, Nightingale was spoken of as the *lady with the lamp* who walked among the wounded men in her care, showing human concern. She was also known as a woman who *heard the voice* of spiritual guidance; truthfully, she had mystic tendencies. These traits and behaviors have been conveniently forgotten in most of the literature in this day and age. Now, one hears little or nothing, for example, of her own struggles between Catholic and Anglican values.

Instead, we hear of Nightingale the statistician and the environmentalist. This is not to say that she was not all of these things. But the emphasis is seldom on an effort to give a balanced review of our founder. Instead, nurses tend to focus on the aspects of her personality and behaviors that support today's nursing goals.

Not just in the case of Nightingale, but in all of nursing's literature, spiritual elements have been virtually lost from the common nursing language. This is ironic when so many, perhaps most, nurses originally were motivated to enter nursing because of altruistic, humanist, and spiritual values.

Even though embedding spirituality in our practice is a challenge, it can make nursing a better craft, a more balanced world of care.

The two vignettes in this chapter both took place at the bedside, although each involved leadership above this level. Yet, if spirituality is to have impact in an organization, it must reach down to the patient care level. Spirituality is best observed in one-on-one interactions.

This is also true about one-on-one interactions between nurses and other nurses, or with other staff members, or with other people in the nurses' lives. Spirituality is a funny thing: one cannot hold deep feelings of concern for patients and none for one's other fellow human beings.

What, then, can the nurse leader do about spirituality beyond her own personal values? If spirituality is more *caught* than *taught*, the leader must be fearless in letting her own spirituality shine forth. The leader must not hesitate to verbalize spiritual issues and values where they apply. Of course, doom descends on the leader who verbalizes values that are not present in her everyday way of operating.

Most authors (and leaders) profess that the values they most admire include tolerance and respect of everyone else's spiritual values. This is about as close as nursing usually gets to a shared spiritual value, and it is clear that this belief is built on shifting sand. Yet, what more can an organization profess when the staff itself usually is comprised of persons of great diversity?

The first complexity in valuing everyone's spiritual values is that, for many people, the values may adhere in a given religion or philosophy with its own proclaimed values and beliefs—elements that may conflict with the proclaimed values of another religion, for example.

So the *mutual respect* aspect can be a challenge from the start. It may be easier in today's society than in the past when religious differences were, in some respects, more evident. But look at the crowd carrying placards outside a clinic that performs abortions, and you will see that respect for everyone's values at the same time may be impossible.

So when it comes to spirituality, we are left with no simplistic answers. Perhaps the most important thing we can do is continue to be sensitive to the murky situations in which it arises. We must continue to foster growth in all our staff by not excluding aspects of spirituality from our discussions just because they present dilemmas rather than solutions.

Admitting this, you will not be surprised to hear me complain when I find an aspect of spirituality on a check list: yes or no. Good heavens, we have *behavioral objectives* for everything. Otherwise how could we have: Management by objectives? Care by objectives? Life by objectives? How can we possibly admit that something like spirituality cannot simply be *checked off* with a *yes* or *no*?

Right now, our predominant ideology is that everything has an answer—a preset answer, at that. This mind-set may be the biggest challenge to developing spiritual growth.

Spirituality becomes more complex, not more simple, the more it is explored. But spirituality addresses the major mysteries of life. These are the things that matter most, not things that are ever easy or ever finished developing.

We should not hide from the complexities we face as a profession. If spirituality always presents us with complexity and mystery, we should welcome deliberations on spiritual issues instead of trying to simplify it into something that cannot be simplified. As Peck says, spirituality is an unending journey.

SUMMARY

It might be a good exercise to look again at Peck's four stages of spiritual growth and think of examples for each stage among the people whom you know. Think of how the spiritual growth stage influences the rest of each of those persons' lives. Learn to see how different levels of spirituality influence the character, intentions, actions, and thoughts of each and every person you know.

The important thing (for me, the writer) is to keep in mind that spirituality is not a final set "stage," but a continual growth throughout life. Hopefully, this is the real message of this chapter.

The secondary message is that the nurse, by the very nature of nursing care, is thrown existentially into all aspects of patients' lives, prepared or not. As nurses struggle to understand more and more the texture of their own lives, so they must attempt to understand the texture of their patients' lives. Spirituality is part of that understanding. Sensitivity is part of that understanding, and spiritual growth is an ever-expanding adventure in all of our lives.

CHAPTER ENDNOTES

Dossey, B. M., L. C. Selanders, D. Beck, and A. Attewell. 2005. *Florence Nightingale today: Healing, leadership, global action*. Silver Spring, MD: American Nurses Publishing.

Fowler, J. W. 1981. *Stages of faith: The psychology of human development and the quest for meaning*. San Francisco: Harper San Francisco.

Peck, M. S. 1993. *Further along the road less traveled: The unending journey toward spiritual growth*. New York: Simon & Schuster.

8
Grief: Part of the Human Condition

. . . joy and sorrow are inseparable . . . together they come and when one sits alone with you . . . remember that the other is asleep upon your bed.

*—**Kahlil Gibran***

What follows is a story about joy and sorrow—the sorrow brought on by fear of the unknown and the joy that comes from absolute belief in religious dogma.

Vignette

As she completed her rounds, she slipped into the break room as the flood gates holding back her tears gave way, allowing them to course down her cheeks. She poured herself a cup of coffee and sat with her face to the wall. Sipping slowly, she sighed. The grief she felt was palpable. It filled the room like a phantom fog reaching into every corner.

Minutes ticked by. A woman opened the door, hesitated but a moment, then walked over to the grief-stricken nurse and sat down beside her. She quietly placed her arm around her and drew her close, saying soothingly, "You poor thing, I can only imagine how you feel."

The nurse looked at her. Her eyes glazed over and sobs emerged in great gasps. The two women sat there in each other's arms crying together for long moments until the nurse was spent. Her friend and colleague said softly, "You have nothing to fear, I've turned St. Jude to the wall. He'll watch over you and your baby."

Being Jewish, the nurse knew little of St. Jude until her friend Rose, a Roman Catholic, explained that he is the patron saint of desperate causes. She had petitioned him to intercede on behalf of the gestating child the nurse was carrying in her womb. Rose was positive that despite the Rubella the nurse had contracted from her 7-year-old son, she had nothing to fear.

The baby was born full-term; perfect except for a profound hearing loss in one ear—a serious deficit indeed, but one with which she could learn to live. When Rose spoke of turning St. Jude to the wall, she was referring to a *statue* of St. Jude—a small replica that she kept in a niche in her home. By turning it to the wall, she absolutely believed she was keeping St. Jude—the real St. Jude— from becoming distracted from other than her request to protect the unborn child. Her belief was so strong it was contagious, thereby comforting the expectant mother. Just as fear, anguish, and hatred are contagious, so too are love and empathy.

This chapter is about grief in the broadest possible sense, not about St. Jude and religious points of view. But it shows how important religion is to some people coping with grief. Dr. Barnum, in the previous chapter, presented spirituality in a thorough and comprehensive way, and we already bridged the cultural divide. We touched on Elisabeth Kübler-Ross (1969) and her seminal work on grief in the chapter on cultural issues. Now let us take a closer look. Kübler-Ross found that when confronted with the fact of impending death, human beings journey through five discrete stages of emotion: denial, anger, bargaining, depression, and finally, acceptance. The first stage she described is:

Denial—the news of impending death is so devastating that the individual rejects it and says in effect: "No, this can't be happening." But in fact, it *is* happening, and as advancing illness and death encroaches on life, one cannot help but notice, and so, one enters the stage described by Kübler-Ross as:

Anger—and the individual questions: "Why me?" Why is such a thing happening to me? As the disease process progresses, anger generally gives way to the stage Kübler-Ross described as:

Bargaining: this is when the salesmen in us takes over, and often the bargaining is with God. The stricken individual bargains for more time. The conversation may go something like this: "God, if you let me live to see my grandchild graduate I'll go to services every day." Or "God, if you let me . . . I'll. . . ." Sometimes, the patient outlasts the life expectancy forecast just to see that graduation. Sometimes she does not. But the bargaining goes on anyway, and Kübler-Ross saw that as people's health continued to fail, a fourth stage was reached, and folks settled into:

Depression: many practitioners who have worked with the terminally ill—myself included—saw depression develop long before bargaining and hang around, coming and going depending on how things were progressing—or not. Kübler-Ross reported that the mentally healthy individuals in her study eventually reached:

Acceptance: and those who did, died an easier, more peaceful death.

Go back and reread these explanations of the five stages of grief as they apply to death and dying. In a previous chapter, we reviewed this regarding something so mundane as a performance appraisal. Now let us review it relative to human relations, in general. This time, think about how you might feel if you suddenly found out that the spouse or significant-other you loved and trusted was having an affair. Might you first feel disbelief—denial? Might you then become so angry you would be ready to tear the house—or your spouse or partner—apart? What might you next feel—depression, exhaustion, loss of will perhaps? Then, if you really, really loved him (or her), might you not want to strike a bargain of some kind to stabilize the marriage or the relationship—especially if there are kids involved? No? Is he or she not amenable to that? Are you going to have to go it alone? Have you no choice? Well, I guess you have no option but to accept this new situation and make the best of it. So, like it or not, you must learn to live with your new status.

By now you have gotten what I am driving at—the five stages of grief are not limited to death and dying. I have found, repeatedly, that they apply to anything that strikes a blow to our egos, our stability, lifestyles, economic security, and other vitally important matters. Therefore, as nurses and nurse leader/managers, it is important to understand these stages and to recognize that our partners—spouses, family members, nursing team members, managers, subordinates, patients, and their significant others, also experience these stages. But do not count on them to do so simultaneously or only one time. These stages are experienced over and over again, and again, and yet again, and when one person has reached acceptance, another in the family or on the patient-care team may still be angry—very, very angry.

HOW DO WE DO IT?

Nurses and nurse leader/managers may deal with death and dying daily. We know how important empathy and ritual are to human beings as they cope with the terrible specter of loss. The death of a child seems unbearable, yet we bear it. A spouse or partner of 50 years—how do we get up in the morning to an empty bed after arising next to a warm body for half a century—a dear friend, with whom we have shared our joys and our sorrows, a beloved pet who has been our alter ego through life's many ups and downs?

Yet we know that if we live, we must die, and somehow, we withstand the grief that we know will come . . . that has already come . . . that we have withstood as human beings . . . that we have witnessed as nurses . . . that we have helped assuage if we have the empathy, the sympathy, the heart.

Death is a major event in all our lives, and it goes hand in hand with grief and suffering. But it is not only death that causes our hearts to hurt and sorrow to fill our souls. There are other traumatic events that we as nurse leaders and managers must confront, and sometimes cause, that will likely produce feelings of anguish, pain, and insignificance in others. Let us move to something more ordinary to examine what that might be. Let us look at something so mundane as an assignment change, a performance appraisal, or a disciplinary hearing. Is grief ever involved in such every day matters? Let us see.

Vignette   What Do You Mean My Work Is Not Outstanding?

It is evaluation time. The nurse manager has spent time and energy preparing appraisals of her staff members' work performance. She has kept careful anecdotal records throughout the year, noting outstanding accomplishments and when staff members have needed correction, along with the results. She has also reviewed attendance records before preparing the evaluations.

Nevertheless, one staff member, whose performance was below average for the unit, becomes extremely upset and grief stricken when told she has failed to meet standards. She sobs and overreacts to the point where it is impossible to have a professional conversation with her. The manager has to end the conference and reschedule it for a later date.

Prior to the rescheduled conference, the manager prepares a report indicating the many times she has met with the employee to review her lack of progress. She had been counseled about these failures, so nothing on the official document should have come as a surprise. The manager is prepared to place the employee on warning that failure to improve will result in disciplinary action up to and including termination of employment.

At the start of the meeting, the employee bursts into tears. The manager hands her a box of tissues and remains silent. After a few minutes, the employee composes herself and looks up at her manager, who hands her the written document. As the employee starts to read it, she repeats her behavior—again, and again, and again.

This continues for about 10 minutes, when the manager tells her that this cannot go on all day and that she needs to regain control of herself and her grief. She thinks identifying what she believes the employee is experiencing and setting limits might assist her in regaining control. After a few minutes, it does. Nevertheless, no amount of counseling helps this particular employee. Termination of employment is the eventual outcome.

Sometimes, when someone anticipates grief, they can forestall it. In the case of the employee and the unsatisfactory appraisal, the employee wastes her energy feeling sorry for herself and grieving instead of making necessary improvements. Then, she really has something to grieve about. She loses her job.

ASPECTS OF GRIEF

According to the National Cancer Institute, there are four distinct aspects of grief. These include anticipatory grief, normal or common grief, complicated grief, and prolonged complicated grief as a mental disorder.

As an existential nurse leader/manager, think about both your patients and your staff members in regard to these definitions. Employees anticipating a less than perfect performance appraisal may show signs of anticipatory grief—as might a patient awaiting a possible dire diagnosis.

Now apply this concept to complicated grief as a mental disorder and you just might have an explanation for bizarre employee behavior after you have given a final warning for unsatisfactory performance on the job.

Nurse leader/managers who work in long-term care are well familiar with the aspects of grief experienced not only by those in the throes of death and dying but also by advancing years. Aging, coupled with loss of function, often brings tears of grief, sorrow, anguish, and woe to the eyes of the elderly. A favorite phrase is, "I used to be able to . . . open a jar, walk a mile, dance the Tango, swim 40 laps. . . ." A favorite saying is, "Aging is not for the faint of heart; it's not for the timid." Those traversing the final stages of their lives make fun of their infirmities, but if truth be known, they grieve their losses and the ease of function they used to have. They laugh about going to the doctor's office as their main social activity, but they would much rather go mountain climbing or water skiing, go swimming or play tennis, or do whatever they did when they could do what they wanted to do.

So be careful what you call them when they become your patients. Be careful how you treat them. Do not patronize them. They grieve their lost youth and you will too, when you lose yours.

Now look around you at the numbers of staff members still working with some of the infirmities of advancing age. Nursing is hard work and nurse's backs and legs and shoulders and hands and feet ache. So give them an extra break when you can. Our workforce is aging. We have many second-career folks in our ranks. Do not make them grieve by operationalizing your wish to be equitable in an unempathetic, unfair way. Some people need an extra work break because they have added extra years to their work experience. A young employee may need to be helped to understand this. So too, may you.

RITUAL BRINGS RELIEF AND COMFORT

Here is something else to think about that you likely already know. It is that ritual helps assuage grief. If it assists a patient and family to participate in a ritual—within reason—allow it. Some years ago, a nurse who was a Miss America from Hawaii danced the Hula in a grass skirt. She did this for a patient—also from Hawaii—as she lay dying in a Hospice in Michigan. It comforted the patient and allowed her to die in peace. How do I know? The nurse told me so.

There is a Hospice in the South in which lives a cat. Somehow this tabby knows when a patient is about to die. Within 24 hours of death, the cat performs the following ritual: he enters the patient's room and stands vigil. In this way, the family members are "informed" of when their loved one is about to die. Then they, too, stand vigil with the cat and are comforted by the cat's presence.

Here is another personal example of ritual that helped assuage grief: my mother suffered a terminal stroke while awaiting death due to a non-treatable brain tumor. She struggled with agonal respirations for 8 days. My sister Mimi and I stood watch. It was very hard to stand by idly while our mother strained to breathe, but she had left strict instructions against artificial breathing devices. One day, Mimi found an Orthodox Jewish patient walking the halls. Every day, he strolled about in his blue bathrobe, pushing his IV pole ahead of him. Mimi brought him to my mother's bedside where she, a Catholic staff RN, and I stood by the bed while he recited a prayer known as the *Vidui*—sort of a Jewish Last Rites. He and the nurse then left. Mimi turned to go for a cup of coffee. I looked at my mother and told Mimi to stay. Three breaths later, our mother was gone.

No one thinks of stopping a priest or a rabbi from entering a dying patient's room—but how about a Native American in a feathered headdress? An African in a long colorful robe carrying a drum? Or a beloved pet?

Many years after my mother's death, as my sister Mimi lay dying, her bones riddled with metastatic breast cancer, her seeing-eye dog Xenia never left her side. Xenia was old for a dog and way past her life expectancy. Her hips had failed her, and she would use the walls as a prop against which to lean to help her arise from the floor. But Xenia knew my sister needed her. She clung to life until about 3 weeks after Mimi drew her final breath and then Xenia went to join her.

Let no one refer to our animal friends as *just* a dog or *just* a cat or *just* an anything. The bonds we form are very personal, spiritual, and strengthening. A young boy I knew who ultimately died of a brain tumor was sustained by a nesting pair of cockatoos and their offspring. Without them, he and his mother would have been less well off. A man I knew developed life-threatening skin cancer. Until his cancer was brought under control, his pet dog refused to eat all but a minimal amount of food. The day the patient got a phone call telling him his latest tests were negative for metastases, the dog started eating.

As patient-centered nurse leader/managers, it is essential that we become expert in the human condition. Although we have many differences in religion, education, culture, food preferences, and so forth, as human beings we have many similarities. Among others: we are social creatures, we traverse stages of life and of dying, we love our children, we care for our elderly, and we grieve the loss of our loved ones.

The better able we are to traverse the stages of grief—which are inextricably intertwined with the stages of life—the better able we are to cope with sorrow, loss, and pain. Thus, we can return to a productive life where we contribute to society, rather than burden our fellow members of the population. As nurses, we serve as conductors for others—we help our patients and our staff members find their way through the jungle of their despair.

Grief cannot be avoided, but it can be assuaged. It can be cushioned. It can be shared.

SUMMARY

In this chapter, grief as a human condition is examined from various perspectives.

- First, we look at Elisabeth Kübler-Ross' seminal work on death and dying.
- We consider the natural progression of the emotionally normal human being through five stages of grief defined by Kübler-Ross as denial, anger, bargaining, depression, and finally acceptance.
- We apply these concepts and reactions to news of terminal illness and impending death and also to other catastrophic events that shatter the ego and the normal way of life.
- The advantages of in-depth knowledge of these five stages and the way they affect individuals and those around them is stressed as a means to better care for ourselves, our staff members, and our patients and their companions.
- We look at death, ritual, and the knowledge that if we live, we must die. We examine ways nurses help ease the burdens of the dying and their significant others.
- We shift to mundane causes of grief and disappointment that result in stages of grief described by Kübler-Ross.
- We discuss such causes of grief as waning youth and function, and the need to be sensitive to the challenges of our aging nurse workforce.
- We turn to ritual as a source of comfort, and the need for nurses and nurse managers to become expert in the various phases of the human condition.
- We examine aspects of grief such as anticipatory grief; normal or common grief; complicated grief; and prolonged complicated grief as a mental disorder.
- Finally, we look to the ability not to avoid grief, but to assuage, to cushion, and to share grief.

CHAPTER ENDNOTE

Kübler-Ross, E. 1969. *On death and dying.* New York: Touchstone, Simon & Shuster.

9

Ethics, Morality, Critical Thinking, and Use and Abuse of Power: Are There Missing Links?

We must dare to think about "unthinkable things" because when things become "unthinkable" thinking stops and action becomes mindless.
—*J. William Fullbright, U.S. Senator (D-AR) (1905–1995)*

What follows is an account of people in health care positions doing "unthinkable" things. As you read this vignette, think carefully about the circumstances and ask yourself why accommodations could not have been made to care for this patient in a more humane way. Ask yourself how you would have handled the situation—and yourself—in a similar circumstance. Please note that the opening quotation from an Arkansas senator and the vignette reporting an incident that took place in Arkansas is purely coincidental.

New York Times, October 14, 2009
Editorial: One Protection for Prisoners
Topic: Shackling Prisoners During Labor and Delivery
Place: Arkansas
Issue before the courts: Violation of the Constitution's Eighth Amendment against cruel and unusual punishment.
Facts of the Case: The patient's legs first were shackled to the sides of a wheelchair during transport to a labor and delivery unit and then to the sides of the bed. This prevented her from moving her legs and from stretching or changing her position during the most painful part of her labor. She offered evidence that the shackling caused a permanent hip injury, tore her stomach muscles, caused an umbilical hernia that required an operation, and was the source of extreme mental anguish.

Although not part of the report, the question is—did doctors and nurses participate in caring for this patient during labor and delivery?

As you consider this and other examples on these pages, ask yourself what you would have done had you been the nurse assigned to these patients. Would you have done as you were told and made the best of it, or

211

would you have refused to participate? What if you refused and were disciplined for failing to follow a direct order? What if you refused and there were no other nurses available to attend the laboring patient? Would you have abandoned her?

Things are never simple, and that is where critical thinking helps you make decisions that are suitable to the situation and that in good conscience you can live with. Also, that is why I placed it in this chapter, in juxtaposition with ethics, morality, and abuse of power.

The previous vignette happened relatively recently. Here is one that occurred a long time ago, but I believe it no less relevant when contemplating ethics, morality, and that third issue that sometimes comes into play along with these others—power, use, and abuse.

Vignette   Do It or Face Expulsion

When I was a student nurse in a diploma program affiliated with a large, full service hospital except for psychiatry, some students were sent to a state hospital for that specialized training. As part of that experience, we were expected to assist orderlies in rounding up patients designated for electroconvulsive therapy (ECT). The patients were terrified and resistant. Some even climbed the chain link window barriers in an effort to escape.

We students were expected to help the orderlies drag patients—kicking and screaming—into the treatment room, three at a time. There we were to restrain them on treatment tables, while doctors placed electrodes on their temples and sent jolts of electricity strong enough to cause grand mal seizures into their brains.

This seemed wrong to me—unethical and immoral, so I flatly refused, despite threats of expulsion. I would only agree to assist in recovering the patients from their ordeal. I also refused to inject insulin, enough to induce shock, into the IVs of young women diagnosed with paranoid schizophrenia. They were a part of a clinical trial program.

Once again, I was threatened with expulsion for refusing to do as I was told. But to me, it seemed immoral to use psychiatric patients as test subjects and to induce shock—just as immoral as I thought it was to force human beings to submit to ECT treatment against their will. (Note: This was before there were institutional review committees and laws governing informed consent.)

I had not yet taken a formal course in ethics, morals, critical thinking, or use and abuse of power. But even at 18, I knew I was being asked to do something that was not right. I did not knowingly apply the principles of critical thinking. I did, however, relate what I was being told to do to the tenets of the Judeo/Christian ethics I had learned at my parents' collective knee and in Sunday school. But as I look back at that experience, I am glad I just said "no."

Now, evaluating my decisions from the platform of education and experience, I realize I applied those criteria that contribute to the structure of ethics, morality, critical thinking, and personal power to arrive at decisions that dictated my behavior.

Let us evaluate these concepts, think about how they develop, and how we apply them in day-to-day practice, especially when the heat gets turned up. According to *Webster's Encyclopedic Unabridged Dictionary of the English Language*, 1994:

Morals: concerned with right conduct rather than legality, custom, or enactment; morals help us distinguish between right and wrong. Synonyms include: truth and virtue, righteous and just, honorable and upright.

In the cases reviewed:

Shackling the prisoner, forcing psychiatric patients to submit to ECT, and inducing insulin shock—the moral test is: Was harm done? In the first case, shackling a laboring patient to bed rails, the answer is clearly "yes."

Dragging terrified patients from window guards seems harmful to me—so I would say in that case the answer also is yes.

Inducing insulin shock—this is less clear. The effects of this treatment were not as predicted, and the trials were stopped. Harm to the patients was not documented. But this was a time in which there were no cardiac monitors available; no crash cart; no codes blue. Patients were deliberately put into shock. What if one of them could not have it reversed?

But instead of playing the "what-if" game, let us move on to ethics, power, and the shackling of prisoners as our study base. If we look at ethical practice and then at power, we will also see that the entire scenario—shackling a person to a bed during labor and delivery was wrong and that *human beings* should have generated personal power to have done the moral thing. They should have stopped it—or refused to participate—or . . . provided needed care and afterward brought it the Human Rights Commission, or some other official body, to seek relief for future individuals caught up in the *structure*, and that brings us to:

Ethics: refers to rules and standards of conduct and practice. Ethics gives us a *system* for judging whether something is right or wrong, often within a body of research or a profession. Synonyms include: principles and values; standards and ideals.

Power: refers to the *ability* to do or to accomplish something. Synonyms include: supremacy, dominance, control, authority, and influence.

Sources of power include:

- *Personal power*—refers to power that comes from within. As discussed in the leadership section of this book, some of us simply have stronger leadership qualities than others, and often, that comes from an innate source of power. Watch children in a sandbox. A child with innate personal power is easy to identify. He or she is the child that is assertive—maybe aggressive. Properly harnessed, that child is more likely to assume leadership roles than her or his more laid-back companion.

- *Ascribed power*—power that comes from another source. It is attributed or endorsed. Example: power of position. If the person with innate personal power moves into a position of power—one with ascribed power—that individual will likely be a stronger leader than the individual with the more laissez-faire personality.

- *Group power*—power that is gained from the faction to which one belongs. This type of power—like all types of power—can be used for good or for evil. Think of collective groups such as unions, political action committees, charitable organizations, social clubs, kids growing up in ghettos, and convicts who join gangs for mutual protection.

   It is important for nurse managers/nurse leaders to be alert to group activities that appear iniquitous to patient-centered care. Street gangs find their way into our organizations. Unions can use collective power for organizational patient-centered good or for their own agenda.

- *Power of the spoken and/or the written word*—power gained through education and the acquisition and application of knowledge. This can be translated to power derived from the ability to persuade others.

■ *Gun power*—power that can be achieved through the use of firearms or other instruments of control. Carrying a weapon to work is an offense that should be followed by immediate termination of employment.

As a practical matter, ethics and morals have been known to fly out the window when one is overpowered and life is at stake. But sometimes, it is important to apply critical thinking to a problem in order to save your own life and the lives of others. A few days prior to my writing this, there was a report of a woman who dropped her gym bag onto the tracks of a New York City subway. Responding to impulse without thinking, she jumped down onto the tracks to retrieve her bag. Just then, a train came hurtling into the station. It was later reported that *had* she lain down between the tracks, she would likely have saved her own life. Horrified passengers on the platform shouted such instructions to her, but in her panic, she failed to do so and was crushed to death between the platform and the train.

Critical thinking, like critical care, is often the difference between life and death. What exactly *is* critical thinking? The word critical can mean serious or dangerous, but it also can mean significant. In health care, when we use the word critical, most people know it to mean that the patient's life is in danger, and skilled care stands between ongoing existence and death. Usually, there *is* time to think through a plan of care—usually, but not always—think code.

According to educators Paul, Binker, Adamson, and Martin (1989), *critical thinking is "the art of thinking about your thinking while you are thinking in order to make your thinking better, more clear, more accurate, or more defensible."*

Thinking about your thinking—"What was I *thinking* when I decided to take that vacation that I couldn't afford?"

Think for a moment about thinking. The word think has many meanings. To think can mean to believe, imagine, consider, suppose, sense, and others . . . all of which are normally done in the blink of an eye—or are they? Analytical thinking is not necessarily instantaneous. First one must consider something. Then investigate to acquire new knowledge. Then one must analyze, apply, and evaluate the effects of what one has accomplished. Sounds much like the nursing process, doesn't it? The fact is, to be successful, one must assess, plan, implement, and evaluate—one must think critically.

Rosalinda Alfaro, President of Teaching Smart Learning Easy and author and educator, in her book entitled, *Critical Thinking in Nursing: A Practical Approach,* describes critical thinking in nursing as being based on the principles of evidence rather than conjecture. Alfaro advises nurses to confirm facts through *scientific method* rather than suppose, assume, and speculate.

SCIENTIFIC PRINCIPLES AND METHOD

What follows is an example of the benefits of using scientific method and principles. It also provides a laugh along the way. I read an amusing explanation of scientific method that will almost make you believe—as did some ancient Egyptians—that muddy soil gives rise to frogs (The Scientific Method, 2010).

In high school biology, we learned that scientific method requires developing hypotheses, collecting data, and reproducing evidence. If we did this with the aforementioned muddy soil, we would soon learn that it is not the soil that gives rise to the frogs. It is frogs in the act of reproduction *in* the soil that produces more frogs.

Once we understand the method and timing of applying scientific method or of thinking critically, we can return to examining the concept, characteristics, and attributes of power. Then, we can scrutinize the rights that accrue and the ability and authority to wield power.

These are things we have all encountered at one time or another. They are things we have all used to our advantage, benefited from, or fled from—things that have helped us and things that, at one time or another, have upset us.

MISUSE OF POWER

Vignette   The Director Will See You—For Sure

The consultant and the director belonged to the same organization. They met and interacted at meetings, and each time they did, the director told the consultant she had need for her services and would "be in touch."

Each time this happened, the consultant returned to her office, updated her resumé and her presentation materials ensuring that they were congruent with the director's organization. She then looked forward to hearing from the Director. The call never came. This scenario was repeated each time they met at a function or a meeting of the organization to which they both belonged. Finally, the consultant bowed out of what she had begun to call "the game."

But that is not what I call it. What I call it is dishonest use of power, and I ask the following questions: Why did the director start this line of dialogue in the first place? Why did she not just use the biggest little word in English—the "if" word—and say, "*If* I need your services I'll be sure to give you a call?" Or better yet, why did she say anything at all? Remember, the consultant never offered her services.

Here is another tale of misuse of power: a candidate for a position sent his resumé for consideration for a "big" job some 1,500 miles from his home. Although the chief executive intended to hire her friend who lived nearby, she had to show good faith by interviewing several outsiders. So she told her assistant to set up the appointment, never intending to actually see the candidate. The candidate called the airlines, made hotel reservations, and hopped a flight. He was very excited but could only share the news with his immediate family because the interview was confidential.

He arrived in the area and headed for the employment setting. When he got there, the secretary told him the appointment had been cancelled. He asked if it could be rescheduled and reminded her that he had traveled a long distance. She replied saying there was nothing she could do and that someone would be in touch. He knew from her tone that he was being dismissed. He fought back tears as he turned and left.

Here comes another *res ipsa loquitor*. This kind of abuse of power has no place in nursing leadership. Some people might agree that nursing leaders who abuse people in this way are just plain mean, but in this case, it was worse than mean—it was immoral. A member of the caring profession cared so little that she deliberately allowed her secretary to lie to a hopeful candidate. He then booked a trip, paid for a ticket and a hotel room, and all that went with it. Then with good intentions and hopefulness, he traveled the distance.

She is but an example. I have many such stories to tell of promises made but not kept; of hope built only to be dashed upon the rocks of despair; of good nurses kept dangling by rude recruiters and disinterested middle managers, even during the worst of the shortages.

Here is another account of misuse of power, this one in a university hard hit by low enrollment. This in itself sounds peculiar considering the shortage of nurses resulting in job availability. But one must also consider the economic downturn causing fiscal strife for many would-be scholastic candidates.

An academic with a sterling and international record of achievement approached a dean of a well-known university. She told her she would like to teach a course or two during the upcoming semester. The dean assured her she would grant her a professorship and place her on adjunct faculty. She would be scheduled to teach at least one, and likely two, graduate-level courses.

The professor heard nothing for an entire summer. As the fall semester approached, she contacted the dean who told her to not worry, she was "on the schedule," and would soon be notified as to what classes she would be assigned. Soon, it was 2 weeks before school's start. She finally reached the faculty member responsible for finalizing the schedule. "Oh," she said. "Weren't you notified that enrollment was low so you were dropped from the roster?"

Throughout this book, I have used the phrase *res ipsa loquitor*— the thing speaks for itself. If we treat our colleagues in so cavalier a manner, how can we be trusted to behave empathetically toward our subordinates, our team members, and especially toward our patients? Members of the caring profession need to be trusted to care.

Were moral/ethical/business practices and principles breached? Consider the facts:

- The dean's promise was broken.
- A legal agreement was breached (oral agreements are generally binding).
- Organizational effectiveness demands preplanning. This was not accomplished in a timely manner. Failure to prepare a schedule earlier than 2 weeks before start of school places undue burdens on students and faculty alike.
- Communication protocol was contravened. The adjunct professor was informed of her oral agreement's cancellation in an offhand manner. Colleague to colleague, one has a right to expect the party in charge to generate respectful communication—the person rep-

resenting the school, in this case. One wonders what would have happened had the adjunct professor not called.

Professor Sue Jo Roberts has been studying the effects of *Oppressed Group Behavior* on nurses since the 1980s. Her article, "Oppressed group behavior: Implications for nursing" which appeared in *Advances in Nursing Sciences* (Roberts, 1983) clearly describes behavior among some nurses that continues to be reported today—by Roberts and others. There is much in the literature for interested parties to study. Just do an Internet search.

OPPRESSED GROUP BEHAVIOR

In describing the origin of oppressed group behavior, Paulo Freire—educator and author of *Pedagogy of the Oppressed* (Freire, 1968)—characterized the dominant group as *having the ability to deny personal autonomy to others by imposing a code of behavior that forces the oppressed down in the name of keeping the peace. The oppressed then took out their frustration through horizontal violence among their peers and those subordinate to them.* Examples include intraghetto crime among peers.

Susan Jo Roberts replicated Paulo Freire's classic research on oppressed group behavior. She ascertained that her sample group of nurses, believing themselves subordinated to and oppressed by members of groups with more and greater power and position—physicians and nurses with greater authority—behaved similarly. A good example of this is characterized in the phrase, "Nurses eat their young."

In 2007, The American Association of Critical Care Nurses (AACCN) in its journal, *Critical Care Nurse* (Alspach, 2007), published an editorial entitled, "Nurses as co-workers: Are our interactions nice or nasty?" In it, the author (Grif Alspach) referred to a paper published by AACN targeting issues of collaboration, communication, and respect. Dr. Alspach reported being "intrigued" by interactions between and among RNs in critical care areas.

When asked about their personal experience with verbal abuse, of 709 nurses interviewed, 25% to 32% of critical care RNs reported that their experiences were fair or poor. In all instances, RNs reported that interactions with other CCRNs was better than with MDs, nurse managers, and nurse administrators. Further referenced in this editorial were issues of lateral hostility between nurses. These are similar to the behaviors that Roberts studied and reported, and that I have witnessed time and again in their many permutations. Also referred to in this editorial is lateral hostility that has been reported as creating problems in Great Britain and Australia. Note: a literature review will reveal evidence of lateral violence in nursing reported in recent nursing publications.

Until nurses stop seeing themselves as members of an oppressed group, they will likely continue to resort to horizontal violence among their peers to gain a sense of power that, in truth, they do not have. Included in the behaviors and often witnessed are bullying, verbal abuse, backstabbing, eye rolling, scapegoating, elitism, isolating, inequitable assignments, unwarranted criticism, and the like. All are linked to power grabs and are inimical to staff-centered leadership and patient-centered care. They have no place in a professional environment built around a philosophy of empathy and phenomenology. Animosity increases and trickles down to support staff and to patients—sort of a kick-the-dog syndrome. This is unprofessional at best; detrimental and destructive psychologically, emotionally, and physically at worst.

According to another well-known nurse researcher, educator, author, and a contributor to this book, *Barbara Stevens Barnum*, power—defined in her seminal work, *The Nurse as Executive*—is "an interpersonal dyadic relationship in which one party has control over another".

As we know, control is a powerful thing. Perhaps as professionals, we should start by exercising *self*-control. The problem is that we are not all professionals, even though we present nursing as a profession. Two years in higher education is simply not enough time to create a professional attitude, demeanor, and style. It does not allow enough time to develop a knowledge base sufficient to place nurses in the same league with physicians, physicists, attorneys, and others who have studied history and philosophy, and ethics and legal issues as they affect health care—not to mention literature and the classics. I will talk more about this in the epilogue. For now let us get back to power.

PUTTING POWER TO THE TEST

The other side to the bullying coin is that some people react to power in another way. I have noticed that even the word "power"—much less the thought of wielding power over another—causes varying degrees of discomfort in some nurses. This is especially true among female nurses, even those in various leadership levels. Power, however, when used for the common good or for patient-centered care enhancement, is often necessary to get the job done. Nonetheless, there are some nurses who have both the credentials and expertise to move into management positions, yet choose to stay put. When queried, many have told me that it is because they have observed that their managers have responsibility without authority—or power.

Vignette A Formula for Failure

It was considered to be the worst unit in the hospital. Staff and patient satisfaction was low. Turnover was high and iatrogenic conditions numerous. A new assistant director of nursing (ADN) was employed to correct the problems. He was charged with bringing the unit into line with the rest of the hospital that enjoyed a good reputation both within the organization and the surrounding community.

The new ADN was well educated and experienced, and he demonstrated a high level of expertise. He articulated courage and looked forward to accepting the challenge of effecting change.

It did not take him long to identify the problems and formulate an action plan. An important part of that plan was to adjust the performance of several staff members. Failing that, they understood that they would need to enter a program of progressive discipline up to and including termination of employment.

He reviewed the plan with his manager and received her support before he commenced. All but one staff member made progress. That one failed all attempts to bring him to acceptable achievement levels, and he deliberately caused trouble among the staff and openly defied the manager.

The employee was counseled and warned that continued failure to improve would result in suspension. That was when the program hit a brick wall, and the manager was emasculated. The head of the department reversed the suspension, and the manager lost all credibility. When the staff learned of this, the manager had responsibility without authority. Soon, he left the organization for another position. It did not take long for things to return to the same sad state they were in before the manager arrived. The broken unit the manager attempted to fix was broken once again.

In this case, the manager attempted to use positive power to correct deficiencies that negatively impacted both staff and patients. But someone with greater power overrode him to the disadvantage of all. The odd thing was that she was the one who brought him in, in the first place.

POWER

These are times of short staffing, heavy patient demands, cultural dissonance, communicable disease, and terrorist threats. These are times when
we might wish for genius, ingenuity, endless endurance, and superhuman
strength—times when *power* should not be shunned, but should be embraced as vital to our patient's (and staff's) well-being.

What follows is one example of how inherent power benefited an entire
nursing staff and the patients for whom they cared.

Vignette   "He Holds Thy Life in His Hands"

She was newly appointed to the position of ADN on the night shift
in a large urban hospital. Upon entering the building for her first
shift, she noticed a large bronze plaque positioned prominently
over the reception desk. Carved on it in old-style impressive letter-
ing were the words, "Honour Thy Physician As God For He Holds
Thy Life In His Hands."

She immediately called for a maintenance employee to bring
her a hammer, chisel, and ladder, which she climbed without de-
lay. Deftly, she used the tools to pry the plaque from the wall. She
quickly deposited it in a nearby garbage receptacle accompanied
by a round of applause. Politely thanking the gathering crowd, she
started on her rounds, preceded only by the story of what she had
done.

Word rapidly spread throughout the medical center that this
new leader was either fearless, crazy, or imbued with extreme
power. It was not long before the staff determined that she was
indeed a powerhouse and that she used her innate power for the
betterment of staff and patients alike.

Soon, her reputation spread—she had established patient-
centered care, staff conferences, had refocused manager's time and
attention, reduced patient errors and regulatory deficiencies, and
minimized staff and patient complaints.

It was not long before she was asked to interview for a CNE position in a nearby suburban medical center. All went well until she
asked about RN salaries. She learned that they were below community standards. To bring them into line and make them competitive
with other health care organizations in surrounding communities,

she requested a $2/hour across-the-board raise for all RNs. This was at a time when $2/hour was considered substantial.

Instead, she was offered an increase in *her* salary package. She turned it down. Shortly thereafter, she received a phone call from the CEO stating that her demands had been met. She accepted the offer and they agreed to a starting date.

Discussion

This CNE epitomized personal power. But that is not all she had. She also had nursing expertise, organizational and communication effectiveness, an abundance of courage, charisma, leadership and management skill, and other attributes discussed throughout this book. She proceeded through a long successful career influencing many nurses and the care delivered to thousands of patients. But the truth is that, without personal power, she would not have taken that first step, and although she did not influence my first step, she influenced practically all my steps thereafter and is acknowledged herein for so doing.

Here is an account of the step I took without her that put me into juxtaposition with her. Did it take personal power to get me out of the box I was in, or did it just take nerve? Maybe they are one and the same.

Vignette   Personal Power Can Pave the Way

I had been a part-time home care nurse for 6 years. I enjoyed the autonomy and independent practice of my job, but I needed to earn more money. The supervisor of the home care department at one of the hospitals from which we got many of our referrals suggested I interview at a new long-term care rehab facility on the same campus as the hospital in which she worked. "Get in at the start of something new," she recommended.

That Sunday, in the health care classifieds in the *New York Times*, I spotted the words, "Get in at the start of something new." I thought, "Kismet!" and gave them a call.

The job was for an ADN. I ignored the requirements I lacked— a master's degree, in-patient, long-term care and leadership experience, and several other things I did not have. I called personnel. During a lengthy telephone interview, I persuaded the personnel director to pass me on to the CNE who agreed to hire me as an administrative coordinator. "After all," I had said, "I'm really the one taking the chance. If I don't work out, you can always fire me."

Well, it did work out, and after less than 4 months, I was promoted to ADN. I remained with that organization for nearly 7 years. During that time, I met this powerhouse of a CNE in an adjacent hospital, and once again, she influenced my life, and Kismet struck for a second time.

The long and the short of it is, I applied for a job for which I was not qualified—CNE of a large acute care hospital—but only by virtue of experience. Because of my mentor next door, I was hired. It was there that I met the man who would become my husband. Had it not been for her, I would not have landed the job or met the man. Kismet indeed.

Here is yet another story of personal power and expertise without years of experience—I have many more, but allow this to suffice.

Vignette   Personal Power Comes in All Sizes

She was small in stature, young in years, and had only 1 year experience in the specialty being discussed. The advertisement describing the position called for 5 years experience. She persuaded the recruiter to see her by convincing her that there was a huge difference between experience and expertise.

In truth, neither the word experience nor expertise reflected the power of this applicant's intellect or her ability to win over the recruiter and make her believe that she was the best person for the job—a chief editor's position with a popular nursing journal. What finally influenced the recruiter were pages and pages of foolscap filled with recommendations as to how to improve the journal—all of them valid.

When offered the job, she insisted on bringing with her, her assistant editor, who is still with the company these many years later. As you reflect on this account of youth, inexperience, expertise, and success, think about professionals you have encountered. Consider those with long years of experience, but who lacked expertise. Now compare them to newcomers who seemed to absorb knowledge and skill like a giant sponge.

One of the aforementioned candidates was an RN, the other was not. Both were skillful in their fields of endeavor. The following story is about several RNs whose area of expertise was critical care. They all were proficient in that specialty. What they had a lot to learn about was morality and ethical practice. Unfortunately, they learned the hard way and suffered consequences.

Vignette Cover for Your Colleague and Cross the Ethical Line

Three ICU nurses entered their director's office. They were visibly upset and took a seat only at her insistence. After much encouragement, one of them spoke. She related a story that seemed unbelievable. Apparently, one of their colleagues had been reporting to work under the influence of drugs for the past several weeks and had been relying on his coworkers to "cover" for him.

This evening, however, these three nurses felt they could no longer continue to do so. He was so "stoned," as they put it, that he was "waltzing with an IV pole" and vaulting over a stretcher.

With a security guard's assistance, they had restrained him in the utility room. The director picked up the phone and called the chief of security asking that he go to the ICU to validate the report, remove the nurse from the unit, and escort him to her office. She thanked the three nurses and directed them to return to the ICU where they were to keep themselves available until called back to give a statement. She asked them to not discuss this with anyone.

She then telephoned the Federal Bureau of Narcotics and reported the matter. The nurses who knew of this all were guilty of breaching their professional code of ethics, endangering patients, and placing their professional licenses in jeopardy. Reports would have to be made to the State Board of Nursing after an investigation was completed to determine the extent of each nurse's involvement. Legal action was left to the police.

Misplaced loyalty is a dangerous thing. The impaired nurse not only endangered patients but he endangered himself and everyone with whom he had contact. Every nurse who knew of his impairment had an ethical, moral, and legal obligation to report him and obtain help for him, and yet, they chose to "protect" him from discovery.

Action had to be taken against each of them—not only by their employer but also by federal authorities. Each ended up having their professional licenses suspended. All I can say is res ipsa loquitor—and W-A-S for What A Shame.

For a change of pace, let us take a look at professional ethics and personal morality dictating action in the face of overwhelming pain.

<u>**Vignette**</u>   **Ethical Behavior When the Enemy Is Pain**

Her sister was stricken with breast cancer for the third time. After a lumpectomy followed by a mastectomy, she had a course of chemo. The toxic drugs coursed through her body and attacked her hair and nails. It induced extreme nausea and vomiting and painful sores in her mouth. But it was worth it, she thought, because the cancer seemed to be gone—there was no sign of it on scan after scan, after scan, and so, she relaxed, and her hair grew back and the weight she lost, she regained.

Then one day, there was a spot on her lung and then one on her liver. The chemo was resumed. But this time, it was more noxious; her heart did not like it, and neither did the nerves in her arches. Eventually, the cancer won the battle, and the only place it did not invade were the soles of her feet—every other place on her thin, frail, body was a bonfire of agony that only morphine seemed able to quench. But like a conflagration that will not die out, the pain became more acute and ever more morphine was needed to bring even momentary relief; to allow her to rest for an instant, to breathe without gasping.

Then came the day when the extra shot brought with it respiratory depression, and a young soul said, "You've crossed the line—you'll kill her with that amount of morphine!"

But an older soul intervened and said, "No, I'm just relieving her pain—that's all that matters now."

And in that blink of an eye, we enter the realm of ethical study called Teleology—derived from the Greek *teleological*, meaning *end* or *purpose*—succinctly described as:

■ *The ends justify the means*—in this:
■ *Intention is important*

With the patient suffering from the cancer eating at her bones like a giant worm gnawing away as if its very life depended on its ability to suck the last bit of marrow along with the final breath of this wife, mother, sister, friend, the practitioner's *intention* while holding the morphine-filled syringe was the most important parameter in that quiet room, where death hovered, wraithlike, waiting patiently for its prey. *That* this woman would die was a given. *How* this woman would die was up to those around her. They had the *power* over the agony that was consuming her. The only question was: would they implement it?

So, we turn to other realms of ethical study:

- *Deontology*, whereby the act is judged compared to given principles or rules. In the above example, the shot of morphine that might depress respiration could be judged by some to hasten death.
- *Moral uncertainty is therefore generated (unsure what values apply)*. There is a popular TV show in which a World War Two Medal of Honor recipient is in danger of having his award rescinded. He is being charged with having murdered a fellow soldier during an enemy attack. It turns out that he indeed killed his colleague, but not in a jealous rage as others believed. He killed him to protect his platoon from being discovered by enemy forces due to the agonizing cries of the grievously and mortally wounded man. Once understood, moral uncertainty was dispelled.
- *Religious beliefs* that counsel against doing anything that hastens the moment of death.
- There are some members of orthodox religions who will not place their loved ones in hospice where life-extending measures are withdrawn. They will not allow that extra dose of morphine because they fear that by so doing they might be hastening the moment of death. They do not believe in extubating patients in vegetative states for the same reasons.
- Morality is not a simple matter, and what seems morally correct to one may seem grossly immoral to another. Think of the emotion generated on both sides of the abortion and death sentence debate in this country.
- *Moral distress*. You know what is right, but institutional constraints prohibit or dictate action. Many nurses have told me that

when patients with no reasonable hope of recovery are retained in critical care units and subjected to complex care, they, the nurses, suffer high levels of distress. Not only are these patients being denied the palliative care they deserve, but other patients who require complex critical care may not get it because beds are otherwise occupied.

■ *Moral dilemma.* This occurs when two or more moral principles apply but lead to inconsistent courses of action. Google moral dilemmas. There are many examples. Read through them and see what decisions you would make when confronted with two impossible choices. Here is an example:

You are an inmate in a concentration camp. A sadistic guard is about to hang your son, who tried to escape. The guard orders you to pull the chair from underneath your son. He says that if you do not, he will not only kill your son, but some other innocent inmate as well. You do not have any doubt that he means what he says. What do you do?

Here is another:

Your niece and daughter ignore your instructions and enter the surf without supervision. After a few minutes, you hear them both screaming. They are caught in a rip tide. You swim quickly out to them, but when you get there, you realize that you need to make an agonizing decision—which of the girls will you rescue first? You have enough strength to rescue them both, but you can only do so one at a time. You look at the two girls. If you take your daughter back first, your niece will not survive. If you take your niece back first—you estimate that your daughter has a 50% probability of staying afloat long enough for you to return to save her. What do you do?

■ *Moral principles.* Sincerity, candor, respect, truthfulness, dignity, keeping of promises, fairness, and honesty.
■ *Core values.* The foundation of an organization or profession; its configuration, structure, design, and relationships.

Example of Core Values—National League for Nursing (NLN):
Caring: promoting health, healing, and hope in response to the human condition.

Integrity: respecting the dignity and moral wholeness of every person without conditions or limitation.

Diversity: affirming the uniqueness of and differences among persons, ideas, values, and ethnicities.

Excellence: creating and implementing transformative strategies with daring ingenuity.

Here are two questions for you—what does the public think about the trustworthiness of nurses? Does image go along with morality, ethics, power, and core values?

In February, 2004, *The Wall Street Journal* conducted a Harris Interactive online health care poll. According to the results, nurses were reported to be the most trustworthy of health care professionals. Also, majorities of American adults said that they trusted nurses (65%), doctors (61%), and dentists (56%) "a lot," and pluralities said that they trusted pharmacists (49%) and hospitals (44%) a lot when asked how much they trusted health care professionals, providers, and intermediaries to do the right thing for their patients.

Other poll results conducted by nursing journals and nursing organizations have been similar. The facts are that nurses fare favorably, especially when compared to other health care professionals. Yet complaints, lateral violence, and other matters about poor nursing care continue to be reported to cause problems within the system. I refer you to such things as nosocomial infections and other iatrogenic problems such as pressure injuries, things we correct suggesting that they could have been prevented in the first place. There also is labor management unrest as represented by a nurses strike threatened in New York City (reported October 28, 2009). We continue to hear stories like the one told to me, described below.

Vignette   It Should Not Have Been This Way

My neighbor recently lost her father to advanced Alzheimer's disease. Soon thereafter, she heard from a mutual acquaintance about this book. She sought me out and asked to tell her story—not just about her father's death, but also about the prolonged illness and ultimate death of her mother. That story appears in the epilogue. What follows is a brief account of her father's demise.

But first let me tell you about the narrator—the daughter—my neighbor. She is an attractive woman in her mid-40s. She told me her story almost as if she were transmitting a story unrelated to her. The love she felt for her parents was obvious in the tale she told. She literally had given up everything that goes into making up one's personal existence to provide care to her mother and oversee the care provided to her father during a 2-year period. Yet, as she spoke, her affect was flat, exhausted, and worn-out.

She could not personally take care of her father because the Alzheimer's disease, as it is inclined to do, made him combative and sexually inappropriate with her. Her only option, therefore, was to place him in a tertiary care facility until his passing. She could not even oversee his care because of her deep involvement with her mother—actually laying on hands, which you will encounter in Chapter 10.

Her father was not bed- or chair-bound—he was ambulatory nearly until the end of his life. Nevertheless, his life ended with a stage five pressure ulcer eroding his sacrococcygeal area.

Was this the result of evil magic or poor nursing care? I know the answer to that question and so do you. This woman was single-handedly able to keep her bed-bound mother from developing a pressure ulcer during a 2-year illness, during which she suffered multiple CVAs. But her father developed a stage five ulcer, while walking around under nursing supervision.

It is now 2 years since the death of this narrator's parents. She is so traumatized that she still has not been unable to enter her parent's home to sift through their belongings and bring closure to their lives and hers.

But lest you think we should fold our tents and run for the hills, here is a story from the opposite side of the coin. It should make you smile.

DO FIRST IMPRESSIONS HAVE TO COUNT?

While behavior, conduct, and manners are all vitally important in human interaction, we also have to look at image. As the section heading asks: do first impressions count, or can we overcome them if they are negative? The answer is—it depends.

Vignette His Hair Was Below His Butt, and He Was Covered in Mud

The recruiter had a 10 A.M. appointment with an applicant for an orderly's position. It was 11:20—he was late. The administrative assistant called her and said, "You won't believe what I'm looking at—step out here."

The recruiter walked into the corridor and saw a young man covered in mud, holding a helmet under his arm, his hair—tied with a rubber band—hanging below his waist.

When he saw the recruiter with her mouth hanging open, he said: "Wait—hear me out—please."

The recruiter said, "I wouldn't miss this one for the world," and just stood there to listen because she did not want mud all over her furniture.

He told her that he had gotten caught in a Nor'easter on the parkway while riding his motorcycle—thus the helmet—and that is why he was wet, muddy, and late. Indeed, there had been a storm reported on the news. He implored her to allow him to clean up and be interviewed. He really wanted the job and felt himself to be qualified.

To make a long story short, that is what happened: Eventually, after rising through the ranks, he ultimately obtained his RN, bachelor's and masters degrees and successfully entered the management track at that facility.

Nevertheless, I am sorry to say that many nurses project an image that is far from professional. Attire sometimes consists of grimy shoes or sneakers, flowered or otherwise decorated unpressed scrubs—sometimes called the "pajama look," unkempt hair, lab coats that need a good bleaching and hot iron, and long, painted, sequined fingernails. These simply do not hold up on their own or when compared with some of the other professionals in health care settings—and some auxiliary personnel I might add.

Vignette They Longed to Look Like Pros

Remember that CNE we talked about earlier—the one who gave her staff a chance to be heard? The one who really listened? The

one who did not take lightly their comments about a cake prefer-
ence and who responded to a request for shampoo trays readily and
graciously? You know—the one who could not only walk a mile in
others' shoes but could actually *feel* with them?

Recall Dr. Munhall's contribution to this book in her prologue
on phenomenology, then try to understand the depth of emotion
felt by the group of nurse aides who spoke with the CNE about
their attire.

Having made an appointment to see her, a representative
group appeared at her open office door on their break time. She
invited them in and offered them seats. They all were neatly
dressed in their uniforms—sort of turquoise/greenish blue. After
polite informalities, the spokeswoman for the group, a union delegate, said she was speaking as a representative for all the aides who
were requesting—no pleading—for a change of uniform color to
white.

It was a time in history when nurses—RNs and LPNs—wore
white dresses and pantsuits. In most health care settings, aides wore
a color selected by management.

Although there was no specific uniform committee, there was a
nurse/management or shared governance committee during which
RNs discussed with management things that affected patient care
and staff welfare. Uniforms could fall under that category. If nurses
wanted a change in uniform, that could be a topic for that committee's discussion. There was no counterpart for NAs.

The CNE asked what had brought about the request and then
listened carefully to the response.

- The NAs had not been given any input into the color selection, and
  they hated the color selected for them.
- The male orderlies wore white.
- The NAs believed that wearing white would afford them status and
  prestige in the community.
- This would elevate their self-esteem and help them do a better
  job.

The CNE promised to take their request seriously and get back
to them within 2 weeks. She then took up the issue with her nursing management team, her boss, and ultimately with the shared
governance committee.

Results

The CNE was inclined to grant the request with a number of caveats. Among them were that the NAs establish a management-approved uniform code, that they purchase and prominently wear a shoulder patch provided by management that stated *Nurse Aide*, and that they always appear neatly and cleanly attired. Also, that the delegates police their own membership. Finally, they were asked to promise to wear the hospital-approved identification (ID) badges at all times—and not at their waists or hips, but on their breast pockets for all to see.

The reaction was like a class five tornado. Hysteria reigned. The RNs, in particular, became so reactive that a delegation marched into the CNE's office demanding to be allowed to wear color if the NAs were to wear white. They were positive that they would not be discernable to the patients as being different from their aides if they all wore the same color uniforms. No amount of discussion about the difference in demeanor, activity, or professionalism would dissuade them from their position or purpose.

The CNE listened to them as she had listened to the NAs and established the same parameters—a uniform committee would present a new uniform code. Then, within the same boundaries as she established for the NAs, she acceded to their request.

Once the new uniform codes went into effect, everyone was happy and looked terrific—for a week or two, and then people reverted to form. The neatniks stayed neat, and the slackers got careless, inattentive, and negligent, and off went the dress squad to spiff them up—again and again and again.

The moral of this story is that RNs—professional nurses—believed that they needed to separate themselves from their aides by attire instead of by knowledge, attitude, and skill. This brings us back to the question of whether or not nurses are members of a profession or not. Dressing poorly does not help our public answer that question.

As to attire, I am not saying that all nurses dress as previously described. But sometimes, I want to take that proverbial mirror of mine and hold it in front of people and say as did Mark Twain: "Clothes make the man. Naked people have little or no influence on society." I might replace Twain's word "naked" with ill dressed and add that poorly attired individuals have little, or worse yet, negative influence.

Recently, I was considering changing pharmacies—until I met with the chief pharmacist of the one I was considering. When I looked at her grimy lab coat, I fled for home. I wondered how much she could care for my health if she cared so little for her appearance. I, for one, did not want to find out.

ETHICAL OBLIGATIONS AND PROFESSIONALISM

Now that we have talked about attire, image, and influence, let us turn it to an ethical question. Do we have an ethical obligation to represent our profession professionally? What a silly question—of course we do. Nevertheless, some of us don't.

Vignette The Three Faces of Nursing

I appeared on the Oprah Winfrey show in 1988. The topic was the nursing shortage. I dressed carefully, aware that I would probably be representing our profession to millions of viewers.

There were four other nurses who appeared on the show—they all dressed casually, almost to the point of indifference and, in one case, downright *punk*. They also went along with the producer's request that they tell "horror" stories about the dangerous care patients could expect to receive in our hospitals during the shortage. Nursing was portrayed in a very poor light—by nurses. I, alone, struggled to explain how professional nurses could and did ensure safety, even during shortages.

I was not proud of my professional peers that day. I knew the audience was "stacked," and callers screened to portray health care and nursing in the worst possible light. After all, that kind of drama entices people to tune in and raise ratings. To validate my point, look at the popularity of today's reality shows.

The previous discussion concerned TV and ratings and reality shows. The next one concerns life and death and asks a very important question: Do you have the personal power to refuse a physician's order? Are you sure enough of yourself as a nurse, whose first responsibility is to your patient, to simply say "no" when an MD tells you to say "yes?"

Vignette Personal Power to the Rescue

The infant was so hot with fever it seemed you could fry an egg on her poor little tummy, which was distended and tender to the touch. She was brought to the ER by her foster parent, who was busy giving the receptionist information to complete the seemingly endless forms.

The admitting nurse took the child's vital signs and found his temperature to be 106°F. She reported this to the intern, who gasped and immediately ordered an ice water enema. This time, it was the nurse who gasped and flatly refused to administer the treatment. It was the middle of the night—there was no other nurse available to implement the doctor's order. The doctor was enraged that a nurse would refuse to carry out his order and threatened her with termination of employment. The nurse stood her ground and told him she had the right to refuse. She went into the office to call her supervisor. While the nurse awaited a return call from the supervisor, the physician administered the treatment himself. By the time the supervisor arrived, the child was in full cardiac arrest.

Have you had enough time to place yourself in this situation? If not, do so now. Shut your eyes and go there—mentally. You have the baby in your arms. The heat radiates from the child's body, and the doc is yelling at you. "Do it! I'm the doctor—do what I say!"

You believe it is wrong, but your hands are shaking, and no one is around to ask. What do you do?

What you do now is move on to the next vignette and think about the last time you were, or the next time you will be, in such a dilemma and remember *your first duty is to your patient*. Read your nurse practice act. I have reviewed it for you in Chapter 10 along with the ANA, ICN, Nightingale's and Henderson's definitions. We will discuss them all in detail there. Meanwhile, let us consider our obligations to our patients and the length some nurse administrators will go to get them what they need.

Vignette   The Power to Get What Your Patients Need—No Matter What

The place was a large long-term rehab facility caring for over 500 debilitated, elderly patients. The time was when federal money was available for building programs, so the structure was large, posh, and comfortable. But operational money was drying up. Wheelchairs and other necessities of mobility were in short supply. The nurse administrator did not find it easy taking *no* for an answer, especially when patient safety was involved.

The CNE was an agile young woman who practiced yoga at an Ashram several times weekly. She was deeply committed to health and well-being—her own, her patients', and her staff. Moral clarity and ethical certainty were among her strong suits, but she did not have the right to place an order for the required 25 wheelchairs without the CEO's approval. She did, however, make the opportunity to influence his decision by requesting a meeting.

Despite her logical argument, he persisted in his rejection of her request, and finally, in frustration, said: "I don't care if you stand on your head. We are not getting one more wheelchair." Almost reflexively, she responded: "What if I stand on my head in that wheelchair," pointing to the sample, "If I stand on my head in that wheelchair will you sign the purchase request?"

I guess the image of the usually business-like CNE standing on her head in a wheelchair was too irresistible to pass up. The CEO laughed as he agreed to 25 wheelchairs, providing she did as promised, and that is exactly what she did—literally. After applying the brakes, tightening the belt of her pantsuit, and folding her jacket over the arm of her desk-chair, she put her yoga training in play and easily stood on her head on the seat of the wheelchair until the CEO succumbed and said, "Enough—you win!"

Sometimes, indirect power works just as well as direct power—maybe better, depending upon the circumstances. Some may call it unprofessional. But how about calling it influence, or out of box thinking, or courage, or humor, or even youthful vigor?

Call it what you like, I will call it success!

But not every endeavor is successful. Sometimes, we have to find out the hard way—that no matter how much power you might think you have—someone has more.

Vignette   Chop Shop Care

Some elderly patients having surgical repairs of fractured hips were then developing pressure ulcers. Nursing ascertained the etiology to be shearing occurring during surgery. An ad hoc rehabilitation nursing committee developed a protocol that called for preoperative, intraoperative, and postoperative nursing interventions, including flotation devices. In order to implement these based on nursing assessments alone, the director of orthopedic surgery would have to agree. Had he been consulted from the outset, he would likely have been cooperative. Instead, he became an impediment.

The nursing committee belatedly sought the medical chief's assistance to prevail upon him to intervene—doctor to doctor. After much ado, the orthopedics chief of surgery acceded, though grudgingly.

Using the medical chief's ascribed power, the nursing committee succeeded in implementing a pressure ulcer prevention program. One would think that these kinds of games should not be necessary. However, where there are people, there are politics, and the best way to get patient needs met is to sometimes rock the boat—but not too hard.

Here is a similar case involving pressure ulcers and orthopedics:

She was a newly appointed CNE and a first time executive at that level. The rate of pressure ulcer formation was both unacceptable and alarming. Along with the department of nursing education, nursing administration implemented a program whereby every patient would be assessed on admission and regularly throughout their stay for vulnerability for pressure ulcers. Every RN would be responsible to formulate and implement a plan of preventive care, including flotation devices, deemed necessary based on an in-depth nursing assessment. A medical executive protocol would obviate the need for a specific physician's order each time a device was required.

Everyone thought this was a great idea—everyone, that is, except the chief of orthopedic surgery. He told the nurses to worry about the patient's hip, and let him take care of the whole patient. Without thinking, the newly appointed CNE said that nurses do what nurses do best—"care holistically for patients."

In shocked disbelief that "a nurse" would disagree with him, the orthopedist walked away.

Many times during the ensuing years, the CNE wished she could have taken back those words and handled the situation—and the physician—differently, because she only had the power of her convictions and not the power to back up her words. Had she realized the consequences, she would have used the *power of persuasion* and the *power of time* to convince him that the program she was recommending was better for his patients. Instead, she got into a *power struggle* with him . . . and lost.

Let us take these one at a time:

Power of conviction requires confidence, fervor, passion, and sincerity.

Power of persuasion requires influence, advice, opinion, and charm.

Power of time may take a jiffy, a moment, a week, or a month.

Power struggle could be effort, exertion, melee, skirmish, conflict, or a brawl.

We know that patients' needs should come first. But we also know that the fastest way to achieving a goal is not always the shortest route.

THE ROAD TO POWER

When I accepted what turned out to be my last job as a chief nurse exec before I went into publishing, I also was a member of the medical executive committee. I was the sole nonphysician on the committee, and I found that the lack of a doctorate caused a power outage in the room. Everyone at the table was introduced as doctor so-and-so until they got to me. I was introduced as Ms. I realized that my opinion was therefore moderated.

I had been thinking about returning to school, and this factor motivated me—empowered me—to not put it off any longer, and so I enrolled in an accelerated doctoral program.

In 2.5 years, I defended a dissertation and was granted my doctorate at Columbia University Teachers College. Now I would stand head and shoulders with the other doctors—or would I?

Oddly enough, by then, I had made my mark and was on a first name basis with most committee members. My personal and professional power and influence by then had a name—and that was successful patient-centered care. The doctorate was well earned, well appreciated, and well celebrated. But the truth is, power and influence comes from within, not from a piece of paper, status, or position—or does it? Here is a scenario and some points to ponder.

Vignette   With the Help of Strangers

A 74-year-old woman trips and falls. With the help of strangers, she hobbles into a nearby store and catches her breath. Again with the help of strangers, she struggles into a cab and heads for home, where her doorman assists her into the elevator and into her apartment.

She telephones her orthopedist, who sends her to the ER of the hospital at which he has privileges. She notifies her children—one of whom is married to a physician, and the other who is dating a physician. Once she arrives at the ER, both docs have called ahead, and she is greeted as a VIP.

When her three children arrive, they are ushered into the ER and brought directly to her side. The usual rules for only one person allowed with a patient are waived—her family includes physicians and that translates to power.

When it is announced that visiting hours are over for an hour, her visitors are excluded from the requirement. It is many hours before she is sent to the OR, and she spends those hours in the ER attended by family and never left without professional attention—much more attention than those patients in adjacent cubicles.

Once her surgery is completed, she is transferred to a private room, although she is not asked to pay privately. Once recovered and ready, she is transferred to an inpatient rehab facility.

Questions For You as a Nurse

Think of the admitting scenario but replace physicians with nurses. Think of the patient as having grown children who are married to or dating RNs instead of MDs. Do you believe that fact would bring the same measure of attention and privilege to the patient?

Have you as a middle manager ever tried to get a CNE's or an upper nurse manager's attention in a hospital other than your own to alert her that your relative was in the ER and needed assistance? How about in your own hospital? Do you feel like a colleague to the directors, deans, or professors of the nursing universities in your community? How about to the nurse executives in the local hospitals? Would you even think to make such a call? Do you think a physician would hesitate to make that call? Would either call be answered? Which one?

Vignette   Demeaned, Diminished, and Doubtful

How many doors do you have to go through to get to your boss? Is the process daunting? If you call, is the call returned? If you telephone a nurse executive not in your organization, can you, will you, do you expect a call back?

The truth is that nurses simply do not have the power in our society enjoyed by physicians, and to make matters worse, nurses at the top wield power in ways that often do not trickle down to nurses at the bottom. This frequently leaves them feeling frustrated, demeaned, diminished, and oftentimes helpless.

How do I know? Because many nurses have told me so. These feelings of frustration and helplessness time and again generate lateral violence described in the category of oppressed group behavior.

Yet among colleagues at the top, doors open, and help is available sometimes upon request, sometimes through peers. There seems to be a pecking order—elitism, so to speak. But I guess that is just a part of the human condition.

Here is another story—not uncommon—a story about a marketing ad that simply ignores the most prolific but not the most powerful group—both in numbers and in productivity. Reading this, how do you suppose it makes individuals within this group feel about their importance to the whole? How does it make you feel?

HOSPITAL ADMINISTRATOR ANNOUNCES PATIENT-CENTERED MODEL OF CARE—BUT OMITS NURSING

A hospital administrator used words in a marketing ad like, "It is a thrill to announce," "Better model of care," and, "One that enhances the care of the patient."

He speaks to the ingredients that make this possible, and he mentions expert physicians and the latest technology. He addresses integrated care across medical specialties and specifies that they work together with patients, families, and other clinical specialists to plan and deliver a single plan of care. He says their goal is met—to serve their breast cancer patients— "those concerned with diagnosis or actual treatment"—with one team of breast cancer experts under one roof, in what he calls a healing environment. He proudly announces that his organization has achieved *Planetree Designation Status.*

Kudos to this administrator for his achievement and his concern for breast cancer patients. But I would like to ask him why he omitted mention of the importance of nurses, both in his announcement or on his website?

The senior vice president for patient care services is listed by name, but that is all. Medical specialties galore are listed. Medical staff leadership is listed, affiliations are listed, and even the library is listed. But one would think that the service that is available 24/7, that patients depend upon for their every need all day and in the dark of night, would be listed, and that patients might want to know something about the nurses who care for them.

If truth be known, this lapse is not uncommon. I recently heard a similar story from the chief nurse exec of a prestigious hospital with an esteemed reputation for outstanding nursing care. She told me how difficult it was for her to attend hospital events at which medical and research departments were lauded for their achievements, but no mention was made of nursing. She decried the fact that board members and her associates from top administration disregarded her invitations to attend high-level nursing events—even those at which awards for outstanding accomplishment were to be distributed.

Do an Internet search for your hospital. Often, there is recruitment material—some of it outstanding. But look for and see just how much—or how little—the public is told about the nursing service and its value. If your hospital can do better, make the suggestion. Nursing usually is the largest personnel cost center. One would think it would have more space on its Web site.

This would be power *from* the people. But power rarely flows from the people, and like pyramidal organizational structures, power flows from the few at the top to the many at the bottom. Refer back to the organizational charts in Chapter 2.

What follows is actual power from the people, but this time, the people are patients, and the patients are elderly.

Vignette   Incontinence Motivates Competition

Mildly demented elderly patients knew how to influence the nursing staff into giving them more attention—they simply wet their pants. Once they did this, someone had to wash, dry, and apply lotion to their nether parts. Nursing administration, therefore, "influenced" the nursing staff by offering recognition for a "dry" unit. All the staff had to do was do what they *would* do for patients who had become incontinent, *before* they became incontinent, to keep them from becoming incontinent. Administration worked up a rational reward system with a representative staff sample.

Discussion

A reader or two might frown in consternation over the question, "Why didn't nursing admin use the power of its position to force the issue?" The answer is, "It did." Administration recognized that an authoritarian leadership style only works while power is both perceived and real. Power must be externally and continually exerted to be continually effective. Therefore, management preferred a *positively reinforced* power model. This works without management standing guard. So they cooperated with staff and gave them what they thought would work over time: a reward system for a dry unit that staff was involved in selecting. This became a win–win situation.

Power/authoritarianism works really well in emergencies, when time is critical. Someone needs to take charge during a cardiac arrest code, or a fire emergency, or a terrorist threat—when quick action is essential to saving lives. The imposition of power, however, does not work well over the long run, especially in day to day activities. Once you have to identify your position as one of power—"I am the boss, you will do as I say…"—you have already lost.

Sharing power with staff and patients worked well in long-term care. How about in psychiatry?

Vignette   Give Them Enough Rope, and They Will Weave a Solution

The place was a small community-based acute care hospital with a 30-bed, locked, crisis intervention psych unit. The time was 1 hour before change of shift—day to afternoon. Several call-ins from afternoon staff resulted in what appeared to be understaffing on this unit—one to which nonpsych staff could not be floated. The coordinator had been unsuccessful in getting the unit covered voluntarily and wanted to impose mandatory overtime, which was allowed by union contract. Knowing the CNE's negative feelings about this policy, the coordinator telephoned her for permission. The CNE went to the unit and met with the nurses.

Without mentioning management's contractual right to impose mandatory overtime, she asked them to reevaluate their patients' needs and match that to available staff. She also told them if another nurse was needed, she would stay. Under pressure to keep from laughing, they asked what she would do. "Anything the staff tells me to do—I am a licensed RN, you know," she responded with a smirk on her face.

Less than 5 minutes went by before they returned, explaining that they had covered the shift. "How'd you manage that?" the CNE asked. "We reviewed staffing against patient needs; one day shift nurse will stay until eight, when an eleven-to-seven nurse will arrive early. With current patient acuity, that should do it," they responded.

The CNE, after complimenting the staff, returned to her office where she was greeted by one of the day psych nurses heading off duty. "You know," she said, "We covered because we believed you would actually stay."

This CNE knew that what that nurse said was true. She knew that when you focus on patient needs and lead from within you will not be lonely.

Discussion

As discussed before, some people say, "My staff's personal problems are not mine—they should leave them at home." It is important enough to say again. This may have been the norm years ago. The human mind cannot just throw up walls around what is bothering it. The existential leader knows that.

Successful managers influence their staff over the long run by being fair and even-handed, by being effective communicators, by both feeling and showing respect, by never being punitive, by their willingness to help out in a pinch and when things are going smoothly, by admitting to errors and apologizing if an apology is warranted.

I have known many successful managers and so have you. They share a hallmark: their staff will do anything asked by them. They also share behaviors—importantly, they address their staff members by name. They know them as human beings with human strengths, frailties, emotions, and needs. They believe and act as though each staff member wants to do a good job—even if they do not. They involve their staff from top to bottom, in creating new models of care, selecting new equipment, designing new nursing units. They abhor pecking orders and favoritism. They are visible and available—when nothing is wrong, but especially when trouble is brewing. Remember the rule—it has been stated before: *they are expert at MBWA, and they have a big sign on their office door that states their name and where they can be found on the unit.* They do not manage by bullying; they manage by helping and by mentoring.

SUMMARY

In this chapter, we discussed morality, ethics, critical thinking, and use and abuse of power from academic and theoretical perspectives, as well as from day-to-day operational points of view. Situations were examined in which participation might induce inestimable levels of moral distress and moral strain, yet refusal to participate might leave patients unattended and in distress.

- Teleology: The end justifies the means. Relieve pain.
- Deontology: Obligation—but—a drug used to relieve pain might depress respiration, thereby thought to hasten death—could cause moral uncertainty.
- Moral distress: Retain patient with no hope of recovery in ICU rather than move into palliative care thus denying level of comfort care and another critically ill patient a bed.
- Moral dilemma: You are asked to place yourself in the sample position and then asked, "What would you do?"
- Ethics was differentiated from morals in that ethics generally refers to rules and standards of conduct and practice, whereas morals refer to standards of behavior.
- Power was described as ability—to do or accomplish something.
- Sources of power included personal power, ascribed power, group power, word power, and gun power.
- Critical thinking introduced and compared to critical care. May be the difference between life and death. Critical thinking: orderly, purposeful, reflective, criteria based.
- Definition of critical thinking as suggested by academics: "The art of thinking about your thinking, while you are thinking, in order to make your thinking better, more clear, more accurate, or more defensible."
- Reference was made to the nursing process as a means to think critically, not only in the patient-care environment, but in other of life's endeavors as well.
- "Oppressed Group Behavior," first coined by sociologist Paulo Freire and described in his work entitled *Pedagogy of the Oppressed* in 1968 and then applied to nurses by Professor Susan Jo Roberts.
- The three D's of power—demeaned, diminished, and doubtful—glaring differences between how physicians are treated in health care, and by society, and how nurses are treated. Included are nurse executives, deans, directors, other health care personnel, and patients.

CHAPTER ENDNOTES

Alfaro-LeFevre, R. 1995. *Critical thinking in nursing: A practical approach*. Philadelphia: W. B. Saunders.

Alspach, G. 2007. Nurses as co-workers: Are our interactions nice or nasty? *Critical Care Nurse* 27:10–14.

Freire, P. 1968. *Pedagogy of the oppressed*. New York: Continuum Publishing Co.

Roberts, S. J. 1983. Oppressed group behavior: Implications for nursing. *Advances in Nursing Science* 5:21–30.

The Scientific Method. http://biology.clc.uc.edu/courses/bio104/SCI_meth.htm (accessed March 18, 2010).

10

The Epilogue—Nursing: What It Is and What It Should Be

No man, not even a doctor, ever gives any other definition of what a nurse should be than this—"devoted and obedient." This definition would do just as well for a porter. It might even do for a horse.—*Florence Nightingale*

To close this book, I will start with a story that should make any person with a nurse's heart feel distressed that someone in today's world would encounter so dreadful an experience that she sought me out to tell her story for inclusion in this book. Consider reading her tale of anguish aloud so you can listen to her words empathetically. Listen to them with your *third ear* as Dr. Munhall advised you in her prologue. It is the least we can offer the narrator as she wrestles with her grief.

Vignette   My Life Was Put on Hold—For Two Whole Years

My 77-year-old mother suddenly suffered a mild stroke. She was taken to the ER of a local medical center—a well reputed university affiliated medical center in which the nursing department had achieved Magnet Status. Although I had no way of knowing what this meant, I saw signs announcing this fact posted prominently throughout the facility.

My mother was stabilized and admitted to the intensive care unit for observation. Her sister was allowed to stay at her side.

At meal time clear broth was delivered to her bedside. Without instruction my aunt gave her sips of soup by teaspoon. Nurses came and went but made no comment. Suddenly my mother gagged and then choked on the liquid. Soon her color darkened and she had difficulty breathing. My aunt cried out for help.

Staff arrived at my mother's bedside and asked my aunt to leave. My mother had aspirated the clear liquid.

That was the start of a nightmare that two years later ended in her death. Because I increasingly "learned" to mistrust staff and "monstrous" behavior by many staff members towards my mother and other patients left in their care and control, I literally did not leave my mother alone during her two year ordeal. I moved in and slept on chairs, lounges, couches, or whatever I could find. I brought in my laptop and worked on over-bed tables, window sills, and bureaus—any surfaces available—lucky enough to have the kind of job that allowed for that. But come what may, I would not leave my mother in the total care of staff who caused her to be more ill and injured than when I brought her under their so-called care.

The sequence of events was as follows:

- Staff allowed my aunt to feed her clear liquid without assessing her ability to swallow. She developed aspiration pneumonia which impaired her ability to breathe, so she was placed on a ventilator.
- They had difficulty weaning her from the vent, causing a trach to become necessary.
- Because she had copious secretions, frequent suctioning was required.
- This became chronic and she was discharged from acute care into chronic care.
- The chronic care facilities were less than ideal. Professional care and supervision was lacking. Unclean conditions prevailed and she developed infections.
- Because staff was below standard and unsupervised, an antihypertensive drug was given prior to her BP being checked. BP dropped to 60/00.
- I was there and reacted in time to obtain medical intervention.
- Because inpatient care was so deplorable I arranged for home care, despite the lack of insurance coverage sufficient to meet that need—I handled what wasn't covered.
- Because a needle was improperly left in place when a Mediport was inserted, my mother developed sepsis. She subsequently suffered serial strokes and endocarditis. She was admitted to ICU and placed on a vent.
- A vent alarm triggered but no one responded. I screamed to attract attention—my mother was fading.
- The nurse who finally came took my mother's blood pressure and couldn't get a reading. A code was called.

▪ My mother was in coma and I awaited her death thinking about the miserable creatures who couldn't give a shit.

▪ Ultimately my mother died.

Author's note: This woman related her story in a flat unemotional tone. She did not cry, but her story, and the way she told it, generated a gamut of distressing emotions in me. I felt the need to apologize for our profession and the poor, unfeeling, dangerous, ultimately fatal encounters she had with a flawed system and with the individuals within it whose practice was also flawed.

It is up to us to apply methods of conceptual analysis to our practice and our institutions of healing to examine incidents like this one reported; to correct the problems and fix what is broken. Amidst the accreditations, and the awards, and the accolades, these shameful events persist. To leave them hidden is to dishonor ourselves.

HOW BAD IS THE SYSTEM?

Just how bad is the system of care, and how long has it been this bad? I have been around a fairly long time, and I submit there have been pockets of "bad" for *all* of that time. For the most part, we have not—as a profession—taken a hard look at them. Also, we have not put a microscope on why—anecdotally—some people fear inpatient care and why many believe they need an advocate with them when admitted to a hospital. It is time, perhaps, to consider things like the effects of systemic problems on individuals, including our staff members. Maybe someone should start at a portal of entry—an ER—and start by considering the impact on patients and their significant others of *waiting* inordinate periods of time for attention in a *waiting* room surrounded by sick and suffering people. There is more about *waiting* later on in this chapter, but for now, let us get back to the epilogue.

EPILOGUES: THE ULTIMATE WRAP

When a film is completed, the director says, "It's a wrap." This book is nearing completion, so it is nearly time for me to say, "It's a wrap." This epilogue is a short summation of the book, a *short* précis—something to leave with you—for reference in case you want to look back and be re-minded of something.

By now you should be able to compare the opening essential factors with the many vignettes. Think about how you, acting alone as a nurse manager, or in concert with your colleagues, can help ensure that patient and staff experiences can be more satisfying to everyone involved. Develop "third-ear" listening skills and consider your prejudices. Think about what you would want for yourself, if you were you in similar situations.

Review the many vignettes in which licensed RNs have failed in their professional obligations to provide services to which they are morally, ethi-cally, and legally bound, or consider why they may have provided them, but only begrudgingly, unprofessionally, or selectively. Ask yourself why members of the caring profession are sometimes mean. Are you ever mean?

In some instances, management and/or leadership has not developed an environment of creativity or professionalism where staff can cultivate their skills and expand their horizons. Communication, collaboration, co-operation, motivation, professionalism, and a strong patient and staff focus have not taken root, much less evolved into strong patient safety constructs. Patients suffer as a result. Here is an example.

Vignette   A Surgical Bonanza

Periodically, gynecologists and urologists made rounds in a Med-icaid long-term care facility. They would conduct annual physicals on lifetime patients and schedule surgery for those who presented with prolapsed rectums, bladders, or GYN organs.

When a new chief of surgery came on board, the issue was turned over to quality assurance, and an investigation ensued. It was then learned that all involved patients were incontinent of urine and feces. Each morning, the nursing staff would clean the patients and place each one on a "potty" wheelchair, essentially a bedpan on wheels. There, the patient would sit all day, voiding and evacuating his or her bowels at will—in the dining room, in the hallway, in the garden. Over time, unsupported organs succumbed to gravity and prolapsed.

The potty chair practice was considered acceptable to social services, family services, chaplaincy services, many of the patients, and, perhaps most ashamedly, to nursing services.

It was finally stopped—with great hue and cry and much difficulty—when new administration took over and a new facility opened, and regulatory bodies made threats. The people objecting included just about everyone previously involved—including the patients. More than 3 months were allotted to the transition, which was scheduled to coincide with the move to new quarters.

But the question is: how could professional nurses have stood by and allowed, even supported, this practice in the first place? Was it habit? Was it because it made their lives easier? Did they not want to make waves? Was it all of the above?

It was reported to be all of the above. It started because it seemed like a good idea at the time. Patients liked it, family members liked it, and therefore social services liked it. Of course, housekeeping and linen personnel liked it, and it had financial advantages.

It continued because no one ever questioned it; never challenged it. Staff members got used to this method. It was easier on nursing staff that did not have to "bother" with incontinent patients and all the sequelae including adverse skin conditions. No one had to handle urine-soaked linen, underpads, and feces. The organization saved money, and influential MDs made money.

THE OTHER SIDE OF THE COIN

The foregoing is an example of poor care—unprofessional and shameful. What follows is a shining example of excellence—it is a story about Jacquelyn Burns, MS, RN, a nurse leader/manager at Memorial Sloan Kettering Cancer Center in New York City. Photographs of Jacquelyn and her staff accompany the narrative.

The minute you exit the elevator on Jacquelyn's floor, you know something is different. There is an aura of competence, an atmosphere of caring, a feeling of camaraderie. This last feature was strongly noted by her staff when they nominated Jacquelyn for the Samuel and May Rudin award for Excellence in Nursing Leadership for 2009. See requirements at the conclusion of this chapter. By winning this award, Jacquelyn brought home the gold.

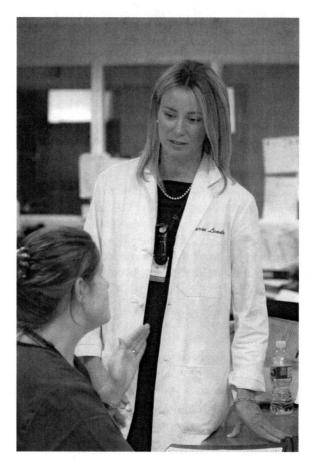

Figure 10.1   Nurse Leader Jacquelyn Burns, MSN, RN, with Staff Nurse Elizabeth Larson, RN, discussing patient care. Photo by Meryl Tihanyi.

Exemplar—Excellence in Nursing Management/Leadership Translates to Excellence in Nursing Care: Jacquelyn Burns, MSN, RN, Unit M15, Memorial Sloan Kettering Cancer Institute

Many of the staff nurses on Jacquelyn Burn's unit have worked with her since she joined the staff as a new grad in 1997, so as they put it, they knew her "from the ground up."

About 6 years ago, Jacquelyn Burns was selected to be the acting nurse manager of M15. She had just begun her graduate studies in nursing management at New York University. Subsequently, she was appointed to the

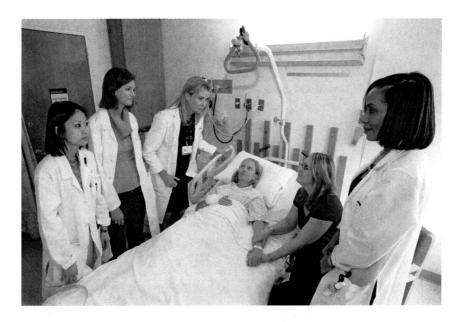

Figure 10.2   Jacquelyn's hands-on approach with staff members and patient (simulated by Tracy Kelly, RN). On Jacquelyn's left is Tara Russo, RN, CNS and Gloria Wong, RN, NP. Seated is Debra Rodrigue, RN, CNS, and standing next to her is Lyndhia Isaac, RN, WOCN. Photo by Meryl Tihanyi.

permanent unit nurse leader position. She graduated with her master's degree in nursing administration in 2007.

According to her staff, Jacquelyn supports their attendance at conferences, in-service programs, hospital-wide committees, continuing education programs, and oncology nursing events. There, they are well known for their participation and professional presentations.

Jacquelyn encourages everyone to develop, present, and implement their own unit-based projects. Her management model of choice is one of shared decision making. Her leadership style is participatory.

One of the unit MDs says of Jacquelyn that she "develops the skills of her staff and encourages them to develop professionally even if it means losing a nurse [to another job]." As a result, one staff nurse was promoted to nurse practitioner during 2009, and seven nurses are attending graduate school and/or have graduated with their master's degree—all under her mentorship.

Leadership in Practice

As an ecumenical nurse leader, Jacquelyn Burns ensures that novice nurses are given the same opportunities as more senior nurses. This results in high levels of palpable *esprit de corps*. Simultaneously, Jacquelyn maintains a close watch on patients, their needs, trends, and concerns. She immediately recognized an increasing incidence of patients with fecal and urinary diversions, and she obtained approval for two new unit-based certified wound care ostomy and continence nurses. These two nurse specialists rapidly became outstanding assets to M15's education and support program for patients with these diversions and for their families. Everyone is grateful for their clinical skill and for their emotional support during a very difficult time.

Jacquelyn makes certain that her staff is up to date on the latest products and changes in relevant and current practice, keeping M15 staff on the cutting edge of ostomy, continence, and wound care, among other pertinent

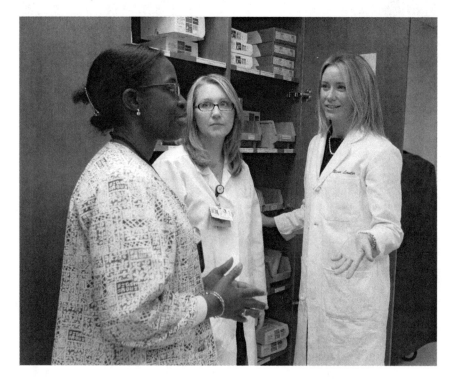

Figure 10.3   Jacquelyn keeps staff members Glendacy Thom, RN (left) and Debra Rodrigue, RN, CNS, (right) apprised of new products. Photo by Meryl Tihanyi.

care needs. Her membership on the hospital's Joint Commission Environmental Task Force has enhanced the important work of that committee. She serves as mentor for several subcommittees, including the shared governance committee—a mentoring program for new nurses, which is becoming increasingly important for retention; a quality assurance and equipment and supply committee; and a monthly support group for nursing staff led by a team of nurses and the unit social worker.

Satisfaction Shows

M15 had over 90% Press Ganey scores for the 3rd and 4th quarters of 2008, gaining them recognition from the Medical Center and instilling pride in the nursing staff. The RN turnover rate was 0% in 2008. This provided concrete evidence of Jacquelyn's ability to develop meaningful, supportive, and collegial relationships with her staff for which Jacquelyn sets the example: Since starting in her nurse leader role, she has been awarded the Perfect Attendance Award for the past 7 years.

Patient Advocacy Through Safety

As Jacquelyn makes daily rounds to evaluate both patient progress and staff and patient safety, she might take a patient for a walk or just have a visit. One of her goals is to ensure that staff's safety efforts are aligned with the nationally mandated safety initiatives through ongoing staff education, increased signage, and strong management support. These include reduction of falls, medication errors, and pressure ulcers.

The simple act of thorough hand-washing is an effective way to prevent hospital-acquired infections. Yet nosocomial infection rates continue to plague the system throughout the United States—but not on M15. Jacquelyn has ensured that signs have been posted throughout the unit, along with alcohol-based hand sanitizer dispensers and gloves, which are now available in three locations in every patient's room.

The result: a 90% compliance rate during 2009. Also, Jacquelyn has led a program to revise the supply mix and overhaul the storage space on the unit. She accomplished this through multidisciplinary collaboration with purchasing and distribution services. This has reduced the time nursing personnel have to spend searching for materiel resources and has had a positive impact on patient safety. Needed supplies are now available at point-of-care.

A second joint initiative has been with pharmacy to trouble shoot and improve the timely delivery of medications to the unit. A forum in collaboration with pharmacy management has been developed to improve medication administration activities. This is ultimately expected to enhance patient safety.

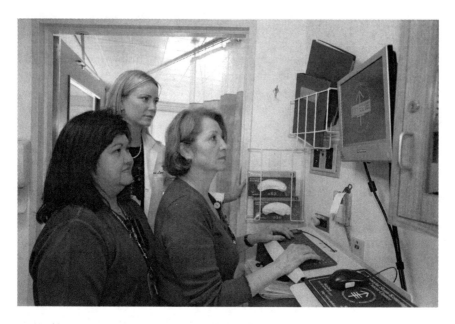

Figure 10.4   Jacquelyn discusses the latest technology with staff members Lili Aquino, PCT, and Carmen Melendez, PCT, both essential members of the health delivery team. Photo by Meryl Tihanyi.

Jacquelyn participated in two performance improvement projects during 2009. Working with the director of patient safety and pharmacy supervisors to reorganize the Pyxis drawers and decrease the numbers of errors made at the point of dispensing, Jacquelyn and this team developed so successful a program that it has been implemented throughout the hospital.

Following this, she worked with the nurse leader of the PACU and a team of M15 and PACU nurses to implement a 20-minute "heads-up" phone call alerting staff that they are to receive a patient within the next 20 minutes. This not only improved patient flow on the unit, but created safe transfer of care between units. This, too, was extended hospital-wide.

M15 is the only surgical unit in the hospital—one on which there is no house staff. So Jacquelyn Burns solved the coverage problem by recruiting a trio of Nurse Practitioners (NPs). Referred to as "superb" by an M15 surgeon, these NPs now ensure continuity and integration of care. This same surgeon believes that this has made a tremendous and positive difference in patient care and safety.

In addition to her hospital-based activities, Jacquelyn is a respected member of the community and is well-known for her fund-raising efforts

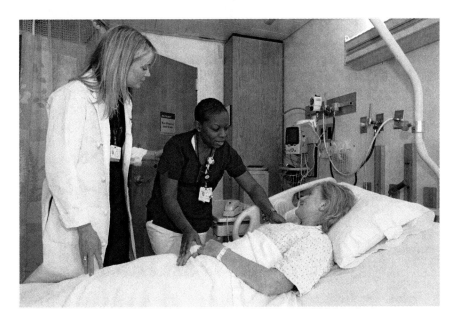

Figure 10.5   Jacquelyn mentors staff nurse Denise Rullow, RN, as she focuses on a patient (simulated by Tracey Kelly, RN). Photo by Meryl Tihanyi.

for children with Down syndrome. She completed the Boston Marathon in 2008, helping to raise $7,000. These monies were used to start a fund to provide swimming lessons for Down syndrome children who access such services through the *Down Syndrome Aim High Resource Center*.

She also helped raise $200,000 through "Tearing up the Turf for Timothy," an annual golf tournament which Jacquelyn co-chairs with her sister— Timothy's mom. The proceeds of this tournament go directly to the *Down Syndrome Aim High Resource Center*.

Last year, an educational program was established with the tournament money to support one-on-one reading sessions conducted by certified reading instructors.

As if these activities were not enough, Jacquelyn was approved for a volunteer mission to Mali, Africa with the Global Smile Foundation. This volunteer group of surgeons and nurses repair cleft palates for children in underserved countries. She also volunteered with the Red Cross after Hurricane Katrina and at the World Trade Center.

One wonders when Jacquelyn has time to breathe. But she takes on whatever requires her attention with poise and equanimity. She is truly a role model for her staff and for those entering the profession.

Author's note: I have spent time with Jacquelyn: She speaks of her staff with the same respect and enthusiasm with which they speak of her. M15 seems to generate mutual admiration. It is my belief and experience that without proper leadership, this would not be possible. As I write this, Jacquelyn is just catching up from having been away for several weeks. Jacquelyn was with the Smile Train in Mali, Africa where a group of kids with cleft lips and palates were given the gift of a bright smile and normal swallowing; of being able to fit into their society instead of being shunned. Jacquelyn said it was a tremendously moving experience—and it was she who was gifted with the opportunity to participate.

Jacquelyn Burns is one example of an outstanding leader. It is nurse leaders like Jacquelyn who give the profession hope. But the question of whether or not nursing is or is not a profession repeatedly arises.

TRAINED OR EDUCATED—AN AGE-OLD QUESTION

The first time I was exposed to this question was in a nursing leadership course in my bachelor of science nursing program many years ago. The argument was whether or not diploma school students had been *trained* or *educated.* The professor had been an instructor in *my* diploma school program. Her contention was that those graduates had been *trained.*

Students in her class—all graduates of diploma programs—had just successfully challenged NLN and university level exams. Many of us had earned up to a total of 60 college credits. We provided this as proof that we had been *educated.*

Educated or trained, professional or not, the issue of ongoing and progressive education should not be a question that generates controversy and strife. It should not serve to *de*professionalize an important industry and keep it from attaining status, prestige, and consistency. Nursing is based on evidence, and evidence relies on science. Two to three years in an associate degree or diploma program, during which students sometimes spend more time in the clinical setting than in the classroom, may leave little time for intellectual pursuits. Critical thinking and the approaches necessary for learning scientific method and other aspects of a broad-based education may thereby be given short shrift. That was why those diploma grads were sitting in a classroom pursuing higher education in the first place.

The passion this issue generates is as emotion laden as it was some 40 or so years ago. Check it out for yourself by doing an Internet search for "entry level debate-nursing." If the energy expended on this issue alone had been put into attaining the education necessary to professionalize all the nurses requiring a BSN, there would be no debate. For those readers who are not aware of this fact, the proposal suggesting that the bachelor's degree be the entry level requirement into nursing was first promulgated in the 1960s. It still is not fact. Nursing even now is not at par with its many colleagues in health care, and while I am discussing nursing's lack of parity, I might add how we let slip by certain roles that went into the creation of the physician's assistant (PA) in the mid 1960s—about the same time as the inception of the nurse practitioner (NP). This practitioner—the PA—with an approximate 26 months postbaccalaureate degree education in many instances has a higher salary line and more prestige than do RNs and, in some cases, NPs.

Nevertheless, some members of nursing leadership frowned upon nurse practitioners obtaining PA certification when it was available to them in some states. All they had to do was pass the PA qualifying exam. By acquiring this credential, the NP/PA had certain legal rights extended to them, such as performing history and physical examinations on Medicaid patients, providing certain emergency procedures, and other things normally under medicine's purview.

Vignette   Health Practitioners Replace Moonlighting Physicians In ER and Improve Quality of Patient-Centered Care

NPs, with their unique expanded nursing knowledge and skill, along with certification as PA's, receive approval from medical executive committee and executive leadership of a community hospital to perform Histories and Physicals (H and Ps) and to cover ER under indirect medical supervision—thus replacing "moonlighting physicians."

The Rationale—Twofold:

- Moonlighting physicians had no allegiance, either to the organization or to the patients, and often were hard to rouse from sleep.
- According to HD code, Medicaid patients requiring H & P examinations in the absence of a physician could have this accomplished by PAs, but not by NPs.

The Legality: The Chiefs of Service—members of the Medical Executive Committee—signed off on the plan. A physician chief of ER was appointed. There were no regulations prohibiting this action.

By obtaining PA certification, NP/PAs were able to extend their scope of practice and legally perform H & Ps and provide certain emergency medical intervention in the ER.

The Results: The Quality Assurance Committee monitored outcomes—improvement was noted. Goals were met.

Some of these same NPs, through the Coalition of Nurse Practitioner in New York State also influenced legislation and worked toward including terminology in the New York State Nurse Practice Act that included the words *diagnose and treat*. This broadened the RN's purview to *diagnosing and treating human response* (see social policy statement of the American Nurses Association).

The opportunity to combine licenses, certifications, and qualifications ended sometime in the mid-1980s, and PAs and NPs went their separate ways—sometimes vying for the same positions. I have spoken to many physicians who employ PAs and NPs in the same office, or not. Some do not seem to recognize that there is a difference between the two. In fact, some physicians interviewed seemed to prefer PAs because they see them as their extensions, working with them in ORs and ambulatory surgical suites as well as in their offices and on inpatient units. Where nursing stepped away, PAs filled the gap. Nature hates a vacuum.

As an aside—by the year 2015, the American Association of Colleges of Nursing has proposed making the Doctor of Nursing Practice the entry level requirement for NPs. Perhaps that is a good time to make the baccalaureate entry level into the profession of nursing as well. Otherwise, the chasm between our entry level nurse with the AD and the nurse with the highest entry degree—the DNP—will be vast. Will they even speak the same language—to the public or even among themselves?

CRITICAL THINKING AND OTHER THINGS

I recently spoke with a dean of a BSN program who decried the fact that critical thinking remains an elusive goal among students who come from a teach-to-the-test high school experience. They have trouble, the dean reported, extending their thinking past the first level. They answer questions but do not go beyond—seeking reason and rationale. They fail to see deep meaning in what they do and therefore miss the importance of individual acts and of their profession. On a day-to-day level, they fail to see solutions to nursing care problems, even when the solution is in front of them. What follows is a story of a situation in which the solution to a problem was in front of a wound care nurse but he failed to see it.

Vignette   Irrigate the Wound to Its Maximum Depth

A certified wound care nurse was frustrated by his inability to both reach the maximum depth of a wound sinus and simultaneously expel saline from a cannula attached to an irrigation syringe. The supervising nurse suggested he withdraw the cannula slightly to allow space between tissue and tip. The nurse mentioned his concern that by so doing, saline would not reach the full depth of the sinus. The supervising nurse then suggested that the force of expelled fluid would make contact with the tissue in the remaining space. Had the wound care nurse applied critical thinking to the problem, he might have drawn that same conclusion.

But it is not only some nurses who lack critical thinking—a physician new to the case removed a drainage catheter from this same wound and replaced it with a saline-soaked strip of packing material. In so doing, he blocked off the sinus. It was not long before drainage—with nowhere to go—collected in the sinus. Soon, an infection set in, and the patient developed cellulitis.

The patient recovered by having the catheter repositioned to facilitate drainage. She was admitted to the hospital and placed on a course of very expensive antibiotics, first by intravenous and then by mouth upon her discharge. All of this could have been avoided if someone had applied critical thinking to the issue—it all was predictable. Another question to ponder is: does attention to data divert attention from patient centered care?

Vignette   Data Centered Care or Patient Centered Care?

Urgent bowel movements and nausea started on Friday afternoon followed by vomiting which continued into Saturday and Sunday. At first both husband—the patient—and his wife thought he had either food poisoning or an intestinal flu and decided on watchful waiting. However, distention and copious vomiting caused alarm and his surgeon was called early Monday morning. A "covering" fellow responded and agreed that he should be seen in the ER of the hospital.

The patient was brought in by his wife. By this time—after about 60 hours of increasing episodes of vomiting, intestinal distention, and symptoms of worsening dehydration he looked and felt awful. He was 80 years of age.

Upon arrival by taxi, the wife obtained a wheelchair for her husband who was on the verge of collapse. They entered the unit and were directed to a cubicle. He sat on the stretcher bed and a staff member arrived and checked his vital signs—his BP was about 83/64, his pulse rapid and thready, his color pasty/pale, and sweat was dripping from his face. A resident attempted a rectal exam that revealed frank blood at the outlet and all hell broke loose when the doc stated, "He's bleeding, we have work to do." But before any real patient-centered work began everyone in sight turned to their computer terminals and entered every bit of data they had collected. This seemed to be the routine throughout this patient's hospital stay, which included a major abdominal surgery to release a bowel constriction that caused an obstruction.

In fact, potentially, his life was saved if you take this to the possible ultimate negative outcome, because his bowel, left to its own devices, would have ruptured. And he in fact received life-saving care initially and throughout his stay. There were some breakdowns in critical thinking issues including more than 48 hours of needless pain because no one thought to ask him if he was using his PCA (patient controlled analgesia)—he was not and therefore he was not turning in bed or getting out of bed. And his Foley catheter was leaking and dragging on his internal sphincter, causing trauma and hematuria—not to mention discomfort. No one intervened for over 48 hours until a relief nurse came on duty and deflated and re-inflated the balloon.

Technology is a wonderful thing. It puts at our fingertips information that advances our knowledge, saves lives, and makes life worth living. But when it supersedes direct observation in a way that alters the care provided so that outcomes become adversely affected, we are in danger of losing our way. So the next time you go to a computer terminal before you lay on hands—think about what you've just read and reprioritize. Perhaps data entry is not what you're all about and patient-centered care is.

As we progress into the second half of the 21st century, it is increasingly more important that we solve the issue of entry into practice before 2015 when the top of the food chain—our NPs (and professors)—are doctorally prepared, and our entry level individuals may be associate degreed. How can we possibly describe ourselves to our consumers? How can we market ourselves consistently? The answer is—we cannot. Nursing is supposed to be an indispensable profession with a unique body of knowledge and skills. But there is too much distance between the knowledge of a doctorally prepared nurse and that of an ADN nurse to unify their body of knowledge.

Recently, I watched a school nurse being interviewed on television about a flu eruption in her school. She was attired in pink, unpressed scrubs, with a stethoscope draped around her neck. In response to the reporter's question about the seriousness of the outbreak and the steps she was taking to protect the children, she stumbled over her words and repeated "ya' know" about a dozen times.

The gist of her remarks was that the school was always sanitized, but during the outbreak, it was better sanitized. I thought she and her comments were frankly pathetic. Were I a parent of a child in that school, I would neither feel confident that my child was protected against the flu nor would I encourage my child to choose nursing as a lifelong pursuit.

Vignette   *The New York Times*, **Tuesday, December 15, 2009: "Exam Room Rules: What's In a Name?"**

This article was written by a female physician, and it concerned—as the title suggests—how we address one another. She noted that while newly licensed physicians, no matter their youth, were always addressed as *doctor*. Nurses, on the other hand, irrespective of their experience, expertise, or age, seemed always to be addressed by their first names.

The writer recalls what she terms the *absurdity* of addressing "seasoned professionals" by their first names, while they—the nurses—called her *doctor*.

Now, you may wonder why I start my discussion about whether nursing is or is not a profession with a dialogue about how our practitioners prefer to be addressed. But if you recall, I also emphasized attire, appearance, and comportment. A giggling gaggle of geese— or should I say young adults acting like girls and boys—can hardly gain the respect of the population they serve, or other professionals with whom they work. Certainly not in the same way as women and men dressed and behaving as mature professionals and expecting to be addressed as such. While we are discussing attire and comportment, I recently witnessed a group of student nurses all dressed in wrinkled navy blue scrubs. Many had on what appeared to be long johns, which they wore under their tops. These stuck out at their throats and under their sleeves reaching to their wrists. They were giggling and animated and all sported ID tags announcing the school they attended—a well-known ivy-league university.

At an adjacent table were several neatly dressed individuals quietly conversing. Their age was similar to the student nurses, but that is where the resemblance ended. They appeared focused and professional. They too wore ID tags, which announced them to be—you guessed it—medical students from the same university.

As to whether or not nursing is a profession: first, there is the entry level issue, and then there is higher and ongoing education. I have spoken to many nurses to whom the idea of continuing their formal education is not only unacceptable—it is anathema.

And then there is autonomy. We have a long way to go before we achieve this across the board. Several vignettes in this book reflect either its absence or the perception of its absence, or worse yet, the stories show a refusal to act autonomously even when patients' safety is at stake. Refer back to the vignette in chapter 1 about the "bleeding wound."

Nursing meets most of the other parameters of a profession— high ethical standards, a discrete body of knowledge, altruism, etc. But until it corrects that long-standing educational disputation— and fixes what has been broken for as long as some of us can remember—we will fail to meet the mark.

Meanwhile, let us console ourselves with another example of nursing excellence.

EXEMPLAR II: WRAPPED IN THE ARMS OF TENDERNESS

Here is another exemplar—this one of a highly skilled patient-centered OR nurse in an ambulatory care surgical center. This account was related to me by a former patient who did not remember her nurse's name, but wanted her experience included in this book as an example of nursing distinction.

The patient was admitted to an ambulatory surgical unit for a breast reduction necessary to relieve pressure on her shoulders and back. Also, she had a family history of breast cancer and wanted to remove excess fibrous breast tissue.

Having completed the admissions process, the patient was escorted into a cubicle furnished with a recliner, a side chair, and a cabinet. There, she removed her clothes and placed them in the garment bag provided for her. After donning the hospital gown, cap, and booties, she settled herself into the recliner. A tech entered the cubicle, introduced herself, and took the patient's vital signs.

After a short while, a nurse arrived and told the patient her name, explained that she was her nurse and that she would be with her throughout the procedure. Her tone and demeanor were friendly and reassuring, and she addressed the patient by her name as she checked her ID band.

She asked the patient how she felt and why she was there. As the patient answered, the nurse put a hand out to the patient to assist her in arising from the recliner. She positioned herself at her side. As they exited the room, the nurse placed her arm across the back of her patient and around her patient's shoulders, drawing her close in an enveloping embrace. They—nurse and patient—then walked in lock step down the corridor and into the OR. The nurse guided the patient onto the table, which had been lowered to a comfortable position. She covered the patient with a warmed blanket, reassuring her that all would be well. She deftly placed an IV into her arm with nary a pinch, and stood by as the anesthesiologist introduced herself and proceeded through her routine.

The nurse was there as the patient recovered from anesthesia and stayed with her monitoring her condition and vital signs as she was transferred to post-op. She said goodbye and wished her well before she took her leave.

Thanks for the Memories

This occurred many years ago, and all went well. But what this patient most remembers is how safe and secure she felt in the warm embrace of the nurse as they left pre-op and entered the hushed environment of the OR. Had she suffered any anxiety at all—obvious or obscure—she believes that it would have been obviated by the simple human intervention of that highly skilled patient-centered RN.

Florence Nightingale, in her *Notes on Nursing: What It Is and What It Is Not*, defined nursing as having "charge of the personal health of somebody . . . and what nursing has to do . . . is to put the patient in the best condition for nature to act upon him." The philosophy has been restated and refined since 1859, but the essence is the same. In the words of nursing theorist Virginia Henderson, nurses "help people, sick or well, to do those things that the patient can't do for him or herself."

When a nurse enters a patient's room and sees a mess, does that nurse believe—as did Nightingale—that it is a nursing responsibility to do something to alleviate it? From what I have seen, the answer often is *no*. The *It's not my job* syndrome gets in the way of common sense and that wheelchair continues to cause a fall hazard, or pieces of paper on the floor an unsightly clutter.

Here is some background for those readers who have not studied Nightingale. When male physicians finally allowed her to attend to the wounded soldiers at Scuteri during the Crimean War, she found them lying on pallets on either side of a trough carrying raw sewage. Her first response was to see to cleanliness, fresh air, clean water, and food, along with emotional support—and as Henderson said, "to help people do those things the patient can't do for himself."

While I am on Nightingale: the reason she is called *the lady with the lamp* is that she carried a lantern at night when fear replaces the light of day. It was then that she made her rounds of the grievously wounded soldiers, some just boys awaiting death. She held their hands and soothed their fears, and for some, she wrote letters to their mothers, and she comforted them. Nurses and others complain of today's frantic, chaotic health care environment—and indeed, it is. But it has been thus in the past as well. In fact, has there ever been a time when it was anything less?

THE CURRENT HEALTH CARE ENVIRONMENT

The current health care environment is perhaps as wild as it has ever been. At times and in some places, it is like a battlefield—staff vying for supplies and position, patients *awaiting* beds, sometimes *waiting* for OR time, sometimes *waiting* for pain meds or to be removed from bedpans, *waiting* to be seen in an ER, sometimes *waiting* for family to bring in food from home because hospital food tastes bad or looks bad. Sometimes, it does not meet the nutritional needs of the patient's current condition. Perhaps a high protein diet is required for a healing wound, but a typical meal consists of rice with a few bits of chicken or the food is tasteless to a palate that is accustomed to highly seasoned food.

If you read through the previous paragraph again, you will see that the word *waiting* seems to predominate. With anticipated reimbursement issues likely becoming worse as a result of health care reform and then budget cuts, we can only expect increases in wait times.

Since the overarching theory of this book is phenomenology, let us talk about the phenomenon of *waiting* and what it means both to people seeking care and to the caregiver. What does *waiting* mean to you?

"It depends," is your likely answer. It depends upon what it is you are awaiting—a good thing or a bad thing. Are you comfortable? Or are your feet in a crowded space and your backside crammed up against a hard wooden chair? Are you in pain? Are you hungry or thirsty?

If you are an ER or critical care nurse manager, do you ever think about the effect of a prolonged wait on patients and others in an ER waiting room? Are there volunteers to see to their needs? Do you ever stop in or take a look into the waiting room? Do you care? Is it your job—to look or to care? Is it part of nursing leadership to look or to care?

If your answer is no, think about the effect on the patient and their significant others once they get to you and your staff if they have waited a long period of time. Think about what the effect would be on you. Think about it phenomenologically. Walk a mile in their shoes. Imagine waiting as a patient for:

- Pain meds when hurting
- A bed pan when having to void or defecate
- Oxygen when short of breath
- Help when a call signal does not work
- Food or water when hungry or thirsty
- A blanket when cold
- A pillow for an aching neck
- Company when scared and lonely
- A diagnosis
- Death to ease your pain

Now imagine waiting as a subordinate staff member for:

- A response to a request for a change of shift, or assignment, or transfer, or any other important issue
- A meeting to start or end
- Needed supplies
- Noncontractual salary increases or other financial issues
- Relief at break time or end of shift
- Promises to be met
- Vacancies to be filled or layoffs to be announced

Stress and tension can be triggered in staff by management; it can then be triggered in patients by staff. In either case, it is likely to generate the myriad of ill effects both mentally and physically that stress by any other means or etiology is apt and able to effect. Therefore, it is in the best interest of everyone concerned, and especially of patient-centered care, for the organization to do everything possible to identify and to reduce sources of stress.

Start with evidence-based analysis and take it from the top. Remember to engage your staff. Use a questionnaire. Finding out what your staff members—and your patients—think is paramount to reducing sources of stress.

THE END IS IN ITS BEGINNING—AND ITS BEGINNING IS IN ITS END

Taken from Kaballah—Jewish mysticism—this philosophy helps segue directly into the next section. It is a summation of the things you found at the beginning of this book. As with most books, this one started with a table of contents. But few books end with one. Before we part company, let us take a look and see some highlights of what we covered:

- Deborah Tascone is first a nurse and always a nurse, no matter how high up the executive ladder she climbs. She tells you in her foreword about this book and advises you to read it. I hope that as you finish your reading, you agree that it was worth your time.
- Patricia Munhall always listens with her *third ear*. In her prologue by that same name—*Listening With the Third Ear*—the phenomenon of phenomenology will teach you to listen with yours. The vignettes in this book and the chapters and subjects were chosen with care. Actually, I did not select them. You and your colleagues did. Years of practice and of listening to you and your patients taught me what you needed, what you wanted, and what you were missing in your practice and educational programs. I

have tried to give it to you here—real stories from real people (including some of my own) to help you analyze how to fix what is broken.
■ I listened, I wrote, I did my part. Now, it is time for you to do yours. There is no such thing as a passive participant—that is an oxymoron, like a giant shrimp. To get something, you have to give something. Make demands on yourself and on your management and leadership team. You have the templates—not just from this book, but from the many nursing leadership and management books and programs available to you. Do not be *meek*; do not be *dutiful*. Dare to question and challenge the status quo.
■ We looked at the Three C's of cooperation, collaboration, and communication. If you do not get it, go back and reread it. This one is really up to you. Egocentric speech, behavior, thought, and action are detrimental to patient-centered care. But so is submissiveness. Repeat these concepts. Repeat this as a mantra until it becomes burned into your brain: egocentric speech, behavior, thought, and action are detrimental to patient-centered care. So is submissiveness. Stand up for your patients. Stand up for yourself. Stand up for what you know is right.
■ Before you segue into the next topic—the Organization—get a head start and remember to assist those suffering from *egocentricity* to evolve into *concentricity*—where everyone focuses on patient-centered care. Use the graphic representation of an organization that places the patient at the center. Then work at melding individuals into an organizational whole, but not by forcing everyone into lockstep. That becomes counterproductive. Individual differences are important. Remember to effectively use personality differences when building teams and making assignments. Work toward the organizational goal of patient-centered care. To accomplish this as managers and leaders, first, you must be staff-centered. But do not accept mediocrity in yourself or in others.
■ Leadership and management are the crux of the issue. If these fail, the organization fails. Too radical a view? Look at the banking industry, the auto industry, and the government. If you want to kill the snake, cut off its head. Harry S. Truman, the president following Franklin Delano Roosevelt, led us *out* of World War II. He is known, among other things, for the saying, "The Buck Stops Here." This is a good motto and position for a manager/leader to assume. The failure of a unit, a company, or a country must lie at the feet of the leader. Otherwise, what use is leadership?

In answer to the question, can you tell the difference between leadership and management? The difference described in this book is that management leads to the organizational goal, while leadership can lead to any goal—even the individual leader's goal, which might be counterproductive to patient-centered care.

- Creating and supporting effective labor management relations take up a great deal of management's time. Consequently, it occupied many pages in this book. Included were issues of contract interpretation and implementation, as well as managements' rights, grievance, and discipline. Remember that patient-centered care is always the goal. Too often, labor management relations turns into labor/management strife. This chapter and this entire book have been aimed at lessening tension between leadership/management and staff. Everyone's focus should be on improving patient-centered care in a practical, down-to-earth, theoretically sound fashion.

- People spend decades studying what I have just covered in this relatively short treatise. If I piqued your interest, alerted you to the fact that we need to learn more, to do more, to correct our errors, to fix what is broken—well then, I have done my job. If I moved you to consider the next topic—personality traits—when making assignments and building teams, then I passed on to you some of my views developed from experience and years of observation.

- Personality traits should be considered when making assignments and building teams. The unexpected outburst from a staff member just might be the result of subconscious motivations. Make Freud and Jung your partners when considering assignments and forming teams. You may hear team members say, "I detest my job. My supervisor doesn't like me. I can't stand my manager. I deserve a promotion. I need a change. I hate nights. It isn't fair. I have a headache." Think about how many of these complaints could have been avoided or ameliorated by a simple assignment change or change of boss? Sometimes, a personality clash is at the root of these kinds of negative comments, and a simple transfer or shift change can lessen or even solve the problem.

- Bridging the cultural divide refers to exposing and lessening prejudice and, in some cases, out-and-out hatred. In this chapter, these concerns are approached in an outspoken, direct manner. This is rarely encountered in professional literature but often seen or felt on patient care units, especially in inner city and large urban facilities. Sometimes, it is insidious and sometimes overt. When extant, it is vicious, detrimental, and across the board on certain groups including patients and/or staff members. When present, it needs to be exposed and eliminated. Reasons for such feelings and behaviors are explored along with methods and interventions for restructuring attitudes and actions.

- Spirituality in nursing is differentiated from religion and handled gracefully, practically, and in a scholarly way by Barbara Barnum. Nurse leaders/managers are human beings, and as such, they often are at different levels of spiritual development than their patients or subordinate staff. This creates conflict. Dr. Barnum describes, explains, and demystifies this topic. I recently heard an account about religion in America. About 75% of Americans consider themselves religious. Of the remaining 25%, although many depict themselves to be either agnostic or atheist, many state they are *spiritual*. When considering the ways in which people deal with illness, religion, and spirituality, the personal descriptions are important.

- Grief—Part of the Human Condition, we saw that loss of a loved one or a job, or even a poor performance appraisal, can paralyze human beings for varying periods of time. Yet we expect them to come to work and do their jobs. Dr. Elizabeth Kübler-Ross described five stages of grief often experienced by individuals confronting terminal illness. These stages also affect those suffering extreme disappointment from more mundane, though life-altering, matters. These events occur as a matter of course throughout life. We used to say leave your troubles at the doorstep. Now, the enlightened, empathetic leader/manager knows this is not possible. Phenomenologically, existentially, this is not possible. Time spent helping staff members assuage their grief and obtain assistance when necessary often goes a long way in rebuilding patient-centered staff.

- Ethics/morality, critical thinking, and use and abuse of power: the paradigm here is that abuse of power without critical thinking can lead to a breakdown in moral behavior. It can corrupt the individual who then can ignore the ethical construct. Reread the vignettes in which individual practitioners were called upon to deliver care under a power structure. For example, a female prisoner is shackled to a bed during labor and delivery. There was no critical thinking to suggest an alternative. The power structure was the prison authority. The moral behavior would be to refuse participation. The ethical standard is to do no harm.

- Oppressed group behavior—*extant* in nursing as far back as memory serves. *Exposed* as a problem in nursing in the mid-1980s. *Remains* a problem in nursing as we close out the first decade of the twenty-first century.

- Question—when will nurses, members of the so-called caring, stop bullying each other and start caring for their own?

- Answer—when nurses stop perceiving themselves members of an oppressed group.

▪ Consideration—might this be connected to lack of consistency and parity in education?

▪ For now, let us get back to the question, what is nursing? For a definition, we turn to our professional body. The ANA scope and standard of practice defines nursing as the protection, promotion, and optimization of health and abilities, prevention of illness and injury, alleviation of suffering through the diagnosis and treatment of human responses, and advocacy in the care of individuals, families, communities, and populations.

Did you know that is what you do? As staff nurses or managers/leaders, as you are rushing around a unit, admitting and caring for a patient in the OR, ER, ICU, or NICU, or rape crises center, or as you are trying to get meds administered on time, while formulating plans of care. As you are responding to call bells, overseeing support staff, and calling pharmacy for late drugs, did you know that you were diagnosing and treating human response and advocating?

If you are a manager, the last time you were quickly trying to finish evals, preparing for meetings, checking schedules, completing health department and Joint Commission or Magnet forms, or God knows what else, did you know you were doing what ANA's social Policy Statement defines you as doing?

The last time I saw a rehab nurse care for a patient —in a rehab unit in a major medical center—she approached the bed and said, "Here's your pill, Mrs. . . . ," and turned around and left. She did not even practice nursing as a professional nurse should, much less diagnose and treat this patient's "human response" to being handed a drug. I wondered if she knew what that might be.

Vignette   **How Can You Stand to Just Stand By . . .**

I remember caring for a dear friend of mine—a physician in the final stages of non-Hodgkin's lymphoma. He was a very tall person and had slid down in his bed. His feet were scrunched up against the foot board, and his hospital gown and linen were soaked with sweat. Several friends sat on chairs surrounding his bed. I had an eerie sense that they were on a death watch—waiting, speechless, helpless.

I asked him if I could make him more comfortable. He nodded yes—a look of relief flickering in his eyes.

It was a private room, and there were no curtains to draw around his bed. I looked expectantly at the people in the room—no one moved. I reached into the bedside cabinet and withdrew the basin, soap, washcloth, and towel.

No one moved.

I filled the basin and returned to the bedside.

I asked everyone to step out into the hallway and shut the door behind them.

Finally, everyone moved.

After refreshing my friend and helping him into a chair, I changed the linen and assisted him to return to bed. I then went into the hallway.

One of the guests asked me how I could stand to be a nurse and handle bodily fluids. I retorted with the question: "How can you stand to just stand by and watch someone you care about suffer?"

Questions and Answers

- When was the last time you brought care and comfort to a sick and helpless individual?
- When was the last time you advocated in the care of an entire population?

I submit that whether or not you are on staff or in management, the answer to the first question should be: *regularly*. To the second question: *in a classroom; by extension; or what are you talking about?*

Yet both the ANA and the ICN states that is what nurses do, and the ICN takes it a step further into the world of autonomy.

When New York State Nurses Association (NYSNA) defined nursing this way:

> The practice of the profession of nursing as a registered professional nurse is defined as diagnosing and treating human response to actual or potential health problems through such services as case finding, health teaching, health counseling, and provision of care supportive to or restorative of life or wellbeing (§ 6902).

I applauded the openness, the lack of constraint, and the use of the words *diagnose* and *treat*. I believed it gave professional nurses vast opportunities to take the ball and run with it.

However, look back at the opening vignette, for example, and see an RN refuse to reinforce a dressing on a bleeding wound without a doctor's order, and then walk away without obtaining that order. Consider the RN giving the patient a pill and walking away. Think about the nurse applying a nitro patch atop a nitro patch as examples of failures to diagnose and treat.

Actually, nurses diagnose and treat human response . . . when they apply the nursing process (assess, plan, intervene, and evaluate), but for some reason, we have to keep reinventing the wheel. Each time we do, another book gets written, and a learning curve must take place, and errors are made, and attention is diverted, and a new lingo for old concepts must be absorbed into the vernacular.

So here is the ANA's Social Policy Statement, second edition 2003, and Scope and Standards of Practice, 2004. It is followed by the ICN's definition of nursing (the highlight of the word autonomy is mine). Until we achieve parity in education with other professions, I submit again, we neither should have, nor do we have—as a profession—autonomy of practice.

ANA Definition of Nursing:

> The protection, promotion, and optimization of health and abilities, prevention of illness and injury, alleviation of suffering through the diagnosis and treatment of human response, and advocacy in the care of individuals, families, communities, and populations.

The International Council of Nursing offers this definition of nursing:

> It encompasses *autonomous* and collaborative care of individuals of all ages, families, groups and communities, sick or well and in all settings. Nursing includes the promotion of health, prevention of illness, and the care of ill, disabled and dying people. Advocacy, promotion of a safe environment, research, participation in shaping health policy and in patient and health systems management, and education are also key nursing roles.

CLOSE: NURSING—WHAT IT IS AND WHAT IT IS NOT

I will stay with NYSNA's and ANA's language—nursing is to diagnose and treat.

- *If* RNs perform these services—competently and effectively.
- *If* they are not diverted by petty rivalry and prejudice.
- *If* RNs view themselves as professionals and are committed to lifelong learning and advancement, so they can climb the educational ladder and safely seek *autonomy* of practice per definitions of practice promulgated by our professional associations.

Associate degree proponents need to finally move off the mark that the ADN is a professional degree. ADN nurses need to put their energy into advancing their education. This is necessary in order to bring the entire profession into this century. Those who do not commit themselves to ongoing education allow themselves to be akin to the journeymen of old rather than the professionals of tomorrow. A half century is a ridiculous amount of time to tenaciously hold onto something that has, in essence, kept nursing from achieving parity to other professions. As previously stated, the emotion surrounding this topic would be put to better use fueling a movement toward higher education rather than sustaining the status quo.

Now then, as my sister-in-law likes to say, "that's it, kids." We have reached the end. The rest is up to you.

SUMMARY

- Have nurse manager/leaders developed environments of creativity and professionalism?
- Vignettes: poor care is described, as are exemplars of satisfying care that included role-modeling, mentoring, clear communication, and leadership.
- Educational disparities between and among nurses create rifts between those with entry level credentials and those with advanced degrees. This causes consumers and interdisciplinary team members confusion. It is past time to end debate that started nearly 50 years ago.
- Critical thinking—Nightingale used as this a reference point—no task too demeaning to her when patient care and well-being are at stake.
- "Waiting" identified as a negative force for patients and staff members alike.
- A review of chapters is presented for the reader to reevaluate what has been presented and to serve as a checklist.
- Nursing definitions from ANA, ICN, and NYSNA are made available.

EXHIBIT 10.1 | REQUIREMENTS
MEMORIAL SLOAN KETTERING CANCER
CENTER SAMUEL AND MAY RUDIN
AWARD FOR EXCELLENCE IN NURSING
LEADERSHIP—2009:
WON BY JACQUELYN BURNS, MS, RN,
UNIT M15

1. **Leadership in Practice:**
- Uses advanced nursing knowledge and judgment to direct and implement the functions and activities of specific clinical programs
- Plans and promotes innovative cost effective, patient care delivery systems
- Creates environment which supports nurses, at all levels of practice, to work collaboratively to achieve unit objectives and *optimum patient care*

2. **Education:**
- Develops strategies and implements programs to meet *educational needs of patients, families, and staff*
- Motivates and enables staff to fulfill personal and professional goals.

3. **Leadership:**
- Is recognized as a leader within the Center and professional community and sought out as a mentor by staff and peers
- Uses problem solving techniques and works collaboratively with colleagues from other disciplines to *resolve unusual or complex clinical problems*
- Actively participates in Center-wide committees and programs to represent the interests of staff and the Division of Nursing
- Effectively leads continuous QA efforts, both unit-based and Center-wide

4. **Patient Advocacy:**
- Facilitates coordination and communication of patient care needs throughout the health care continuum
- Role models ethical principles in the delivery of patient care
- Promotes principles supporting patient safety.

5. Professional Image:
- Promotes a positive image of self, unit, and MSKCC
- Motivates peers and promotes a team environment
- Supports research initiatives of MSKCC through education, practice, and leadership
- Participates in professional activities inside and outside of MSKCC

6. Summary:
  Please describe why you chose to nominate this employee for the Excellence in Nursing Leadership Award:

CHAPTER ENDNOTES

American Nurses Association. 2003. *Nursing's Social Policy Statement*. 2nd ed. Silver Springs, MD: American Nurses Association.

American Nurses Association. 2004. Nursing Administration: Scope & Standards of Practice, pp. 6 & 7. Silver Springs, MD: American Nurses Association.

Dossey, B. M., L. C. Selanders, D. Beck, and A. Attewell. 2005. *Florence Nightingale today: Healing, leadership, global action*. Silver Spring, MD: American Nurses Publishing.

Nightingale, F. 1969. *Notes on nursing: What it is and what it is not*. New York: Dover Publications Inc.

Role of the Professional Nurse Regarding Patient Education. http://www.nysna.org/practice/positions/position25.htm (accessed December 28, 2009).

Bibliography

American Nurses Association. 2001. *Code of ethics with interpretive statement*. Silver Springs, MD: American Nurses Association.

American Nurses Association. 2009. Nursing Administration: Scope & Standards of Practice. *ANCC Magnet Recognition Program*. Silver Springs, MD: American Nurses Association.

Barnum, B. 2003. *Spirituality in nursing from traditional to new age*, 2nd ed. New York: Springer Publishing Company.

Brooks, D. "The End of Philosophy." *New York Times*, April 6, 2009. http://www.nytimes.com/.

Carroll, L. 1865. *Through the looking glass*. London, England: MacMillan & Sons.

Charismatic Leadership Theory. http://business.nmsu.edu/~dboje/teaching/338/charisma.htm (accessed May 25, 2010).

Dossey, B. M., L. C. Selanders, D. Beck, and A. Attewell. 2005. *Florence Nightingale today: Healing, leadership, global action*. Silver Spring, MD: American Nurses Publishing.

Duffy, M. 2009. Preventing workplace mobbing and bullying with effective organizational consultation, policies and legislation. *Consulting Psychology Journal: Practice and Research* 61(3):242–262.

Forman, H. and G. Davis. 2002. The anatomy of a union campaign. *JONA* 32(9):444–447.

Forman, H. and H. Krauss. 2003. Decertification: Management's role when employees rethink unionization. *JONA* 33(6):313–316.

Forman, H. and F. Merrick. 2003a. Discipline: Learning the rules of the management high road. *JONA* 33(2):65–67.

Forman, H. and F. Merrick. 2003b. Grievances and complaints: Valuable tools for management and for staff. *JONA* 33(3):136–138.

Forman, H. and T. Powell. 2003a. Management rights. *JONA* 33(1):7–9.

Forman, H. and T. Powell. 2003b. Union-management cooperation. *JONA* 33(12):621–623.

Fowler, J. W. 1981. *Stages of faith: The psychology of human development and the quest for meaning*. San Francisco: Harper San Francisco.

Freire, P. 1999. *Pedagogy of the oppressed*, 3rd ed. New York: Continuum Publishing Co.

Gibbs, J. R. 1961. Defensive communication. *Journal of Communication* 2(3):143.

Haney, W. V. 1973. *Communication and organizational behavior text and cases*, 3rd ed. Homewood, IL: Richard D. Irwin, Inc.

Hersey, P. and K. H. Blanchard. 1969. *Management of organizational behavior*. Englewood Cliffs, NJ: Prentice Hall.

Huber, D. L. 2006. *Leadership & nursing care management*, 3rd ed. Philadelphia: Saunders Elsevier.

Huxley, J. H. 1982. In: L. Dossey, *Time, space and medicine*. Colorado: Shambhala.

Jewish Virtual Library. www.jewishvirtuallibrary.org/ A division of the American–Israeli Cooperative Enterprise.

King, S. 2000. *On writing.* New York: Scribner.

Koloroutis, M. (Ed.) 2004. *Relationship-based care. A model for transforming practice.* Minneapolis, MN: Creative Health Management.

Lamb-Deans, D. 2009. *Organizational behavior—Introduction.* Ithaca, NY: Catherwood Library, Cornell University ILR School.

Lee Roger A & History Guide Media. 2008–2009. Arab-Israel Wars: Gaza War. www.historyguy.com/gaza_war.htm (accessed May 25, 2010).

Machiavelli, N. 1532. *The prince.* Florence, Italy: Antonio Blado d'Asola.

Maslow, A. H. 1970. *Motivation and personality,* 2nd ed. New York: Harper and Row.

McGregor, D. 1960. *The human side of enterprise.* New York: McGraw Hill.

Nightingale, F. 1969. *Notes on nursing: What it is and what it is not.* New York: Dover Publications Inc.

North American Nursing Diagnosis Association. 2005. *Nursing diagnoses: Definitions and classification.* Philadelphia, PA: NANDA International.

Ouchi, W. G. 1981. *Theory Z—The M form society.* New York: Avon Books.

Peck, M. S. 1993. *Further along the road less traveled: The unending journey toward spiritual growth.* New York: Simon & Schuster.

Peters, T. J. and R. H. Waterman. 1982. *In search of excellence.* New York: Harper Collins.

Petty, T. 1994. *Tom Petty Wildflowers,* CD. Burbank, CA: Warner Brothers Records.

Reilly, D. L. California Employment Investigation Lawyer & Attorney. "No Right to Representation for Accused Nonunion Employees in Workplace Investigations—But for How Long?" http:www.workplaceinvestigationblog.com (accessed December 14, 2009).

Roberts, S. J. 1983. Oppressed group behavior: Implications for nursing. *Advances in Nursing Science* 5:21–30.

Role of the Professional Nurse Regarding Patient Education. http://www.nysna.org/practice/positions/position25.htm (accessed December 28, 2009).

Rosalinda, A.-L. 1995. *Critical thinking in nursing: A practical approach.* Philadelphia: W. B. Saunders.

Spiritual Psychology. http://www.universityofsantamonica.edu/Globals/contact.html. University of Santa Monica, 2107 Wilshire Blvd., Santa Monica, CA 90403.

Smith, H. 1978. *Great religions of the world.* National Geographic Book Service, Krister Stendahl.

Steenbarger, B. 2009. *Four pillars of psychological well-being.* http://traderfeed.blogspot.com/2009/05/four-pillars-of-psychological-well.html (accessed March 24, 2010).

Stevens, B. J. 1985. *The nurse as executive,* 3rd ed. Rockville, MD: Aspen Publishers.

Thomas and Kilman Conflict Mode Instrument. http://www.kilmann.com/conflict.html (accessed December 14, 2009).

INDEX